NEURODEVELOPMENTAL DISEASES -
LABORATORY AND CLINICAL RESEARCH

THE COMBATING AUTISM ACT

ELEMENTS, FUNDING AND ANALYSES

NEURODEVELOPMENTAL DISEASES - LABORATORY AND CLINICAL RESEARCH

Additional books in this series can be found on Nova's website under the Series tab.

Additional e-books in this series can be found on Nova's website under the e-book tab.

NEURODEVELOPMENTAL DISEASES - LABORATORY AND CLINICAL RESEARCH

THE COMBATING AUTISM ACT

ELEMENTS, FUNDING AND ANALYSES

DERYCK HARLOW
EDITOR

nova publishers
New York

For permission to use material from this book please contact us:
Telephone 631-231-7269; Fax 631-231-8175
Web Site: http://www.novapublishers.com

Library of Congress Cataloging-in-Publication Data

ISBN: 978-1-63321-128-5

Published by Nova Science Publishers, Inc. † New York

CONTENTS

PREFACE

This book presents an overview of the Combating Autism Act and Combating Autism Reauthorization Act, the Department of Health and Human Services funding, other federal activities related to autism, and selected issues for Congress. It also describes the actions that HHS agencies have taken as a result of the CAA; examines the oversight of CAA grantees; analyzes the extent to which federal agencies fund potentially duplicative autism research; and assesses the extent to which IACC and agencies coordinate and monitor federal autism activities.

Chapter 1 – Autism spectrum disorder (ASD) and autism are general terms for a group of developmental disabilities that cause impairments in social skills and communication, and are often characterized by certain atypical behaviors. The federal government has a role in the financing (through Medicaid and State Children's Health Insurance Programs) and delivery (through funding of developmental disabilities programming in schools, Title V Maternal and Child Health funding, and other sources) of treatment for ASD. The number of autism cases and their appropriate diagnosis and treatment affect federal and state expenditures. As such, Congress has shown interest in financing research on ASD prevalence, causes, and optimal treatment for individuals with ASD. On September 26, 2011, the 112th Congress passed the Combating Autism Reauthorization Act (CARA, P.L. 112-32), which reauthorized funding for autism research authorized under the Combating Autism Act of 2006 (CAA, P.L. 109-416). The CAA was enacted to address public and congressional concern with growing rates of autism; to increase existing autism research funding authorizations; and to stimulate state-level coordination of health, education, and disability programs. The CAA authorizes funding for ASD surveillance, research, and education at the Department of Health and Human Services (HHS), at the

Centers for Disease Control and Prevention (CDC), the Health Resources and Services Administration (HRSA), and the National Institutes of Health (NIH). The CAA authorizes funding for CDC to administer a grant program for states and other entities to conduct surveillance on ASD and developmental disabilities, and to establish regional centers of excellence in ASD epidemiology. The CAA also authorizes funding for HRSA to support autism education, intervention, and early detection. NIH is authorized under the CAA to conduct and fund basic scientific research on autism and other developmental disabilities. In addition, NIH is tasked with the coordination of all research, screening, intervention, and education efforts through the Interagency Autism Coordinating Committee. The Combating Autism Act authorized appropriations for these activities from FY2007 through FY2011. The Combating Autism Reauthorization Act of 2011 extends authorizations of appropriations at FY2011 levels for FY2012 through FY2014. Funding for research authorized by CARA is discretionary and subject to the annual appropriations process. Full-year appropriations for FY2013 have yet to be enacted. However, a six-month government-wide continuing resolution (CR) was signed into law on September 28, 2012 (P.L. 112-175), which generally maintained funding for discretionary programs at their FY2012 levels, increased by 0.612%. This report presents an overview of the CAA and CARA, HHS funding and activities under the CAA and CARA for FY2007 through FY2013, other federal activities related to autism, and selected issues for Congress.

Chapter 2 – CDC considers autism to be an important public health concern. In 2012, CDC reported that an estimated 1 in 88 children in the United States has been identified as having autism— a 23 percent increase from its estimate of 1 in 110 reported in 2009. Autism is a developmental disorder involving communication and social impairment. Symptoms usually become evident in early childhood. There are many suspected causes and no known cure. HHS agencies fund educational and support services for individuals diagnosed with autism and fund research in a variety of areas, such as identifying the causes of autism and intervention options. The CAA amended sections of the Children's Health Act of 2000 related to autism and established new requirements. The CAA, enacted in December 2006, authorized the expansion of HHS's activities related to autism research, surveillance, prevention, intervention, and education through fiscal year 2011. The CAA authorized, but did not appropriate, federal funding to carry out these activities. In this report, GAO (1) describes the actions that HHS agencies have taken as a result of the CAA, and (2) examines the oversight of

CAA grantees. To address these objectives, GAO reviewed CAA and HHS documents and interviewed agency officials to identify the autism activities resulting from the CAA. GAO also determined the amount certain HHS agencies spent on autism activities from fiscal year 2006—prior to the CAA—through fiscal year 2011. In addition, GAO reviewed files for a random sample of CAA grantees to examine oversight from 2008 to 2011.

Chapter 3 – Autism—a developmental disorder involving communication and social impairment—is an important public health concern. From fiscal years 2008 through 2012, 12 federal agencies awarded at least $1.4 billion to support autism research and other autism-related activities. The CAA directed the IACC to coordinate HHS autism activities and monitor all federal autism activities. It also required the IACC to develop and annually update a strategic plan for autism research. This plan is organized into 7 research areas that contain specific objectives. GAO was asked to examine federal autism efforts. In this report, GAO (1) analyzes the extent to which federal agencies fund potentially duplicative autism research, and (2) assesses the extent to which IACC and agencies coordinate and monitor federal autism activities. GAO analyzed agencies' data and documents, and interviewed federal agency officials and select nonfederal IACC members.

In: The Combating Autism Act
Editor: Deryck Harlow
ISBN: 978-1-63321-128-5

Chapter 1

THE COMBATING AUTISM ACT: OVERVIEW AND FUNDING*

Amalia K. Corby-Edwards

SUMMARY

Autism spectrum disorder (ASD) and autism are general terms for a group of developmental disabilities that cause impairments in social skills and communication, and are often characterized by certain atypical behaviors. The federal government has a role in the financing (through Medicaid and State Children's Health Insurance Programs) and delivery (through funding of developmental disabilities programming in schools, Title V Maternal and Child Health funding, and other sources) of treatment for ASD. The number of autism cases and their appropriate diagnosis and treatment affect federal and state expenditures. As such, Congress has shown interest in financing research on ASD prevalence, causes, and optimal treatment for individuals with ASD.

On September 26, 2011, the 112th Congress passed the Combating Autism Reauthorization Act (CARA, P.L. 112-32), which reauthorized funding for autism research authorized under the Combating Autism Act of 2006 (CAA, P.L. 109-416). The CAA was enacted to address public and congressional concern with growing rates of autism; to increase existing autism research funding authorizations; and to stimulate state-level coordination of health, education, and disability programs. The

* This is an edited, reformatted and augmented version of Congressional Research Service Publication, No. R42369, dated December 27, 2012.

CAA authorizes funding for ASD surveillance, research, and education at the Department of Health and Human Services (HHS), at the Centers for Disease Control and Prevention (CDC), the Health Resources and Services Administration (HRSA), and the National Institutes of Health (NIH).

The CAA authorizes funding for CDC to administer a grant program for states and other entities to conduct surveillance on ASD and developmental disabilities, and to establish regional centers of excellence in ASD epidemiology. The CAA also authorizes funding for HRSA to support autism education, intervention, and early detection. NIH is authorized under the CAA to conduct and fund basic scientific research on autism and other developmental disabilities. In addition, NIH is tasked with the coordination of all research, screening, intervention, and education efforts through the Interagency Autism Coordinating Committee.

The Combating Autism Act authorized appropriations for these activities from FY2007 through FY2011. The Combating Autism Reauthorization Act of 2011 extends authorizations of appropriations at FY2011 levels for FY2012 through FY2014. Funding for research authorized by CARA is discretionary and subject to the annual appropriations process. Full-year appropriations for FY2013 have yet to be enacted. However, a six-month government-wide continuing resolution (CR) was signed into law on September 28, 2012 (P.L. 112-175), which generally maintained funding for discretionary programs at their FY2012 levels, increased by 0.612%.

This report presents an overview of the CAA and CARA, HHS funding and activities under the CAA and CARA for FY2007 through FY2013, other federal activities related to autism, and selected issues for Congress.

INTRODUCTION

Autism spectrum disorder (ASD) and autism are general terms for a group of developmental disabilities that cause impairments in social skills and communication, and are often characterized by certain atypical behaviors.[1] Autism spectrum disorders include autistic disorder, Asperger disorder, and pervasive developmental disorder-not otherwise specified.[2] These conditions have overlapping symptoms that differ in terms of onset, severity, and nature. ASDs are referred to as "spectrum disorders" because they encompass a range of behaviorally defined conditions. The complex nature of these conditions creates diagnostic challenges; there are no consistent genetic[3] or biologic markers[4] to facilitate diagnosis.

Autism has been linked to abnormal biology and chemistry in the brain; however, the cause or causes of these abnormalities remain unknown. According to the Centers for Disease Control and Prevention (CDC), as many as 1 in 110 eight-year-olds currently have an autism spectrum disorder, with boys affected more than four times as often as girls.[5] This represents an increase from past autism rates, and has generated public interest in the causes of autism. The increased prevalence has also focused attention on the demand for effective treatment and support services for individuals with these conditions. In addition, some have questioned whether the current rates of ASD reflect increased awareness and diagnosis, a true increase in the incidence of ASD, or a combination of these factors.[6]

For many, autism is a lifelong illness whose symptoms often manifest before age three. Autistic children and adults generally display a unique set of symptoms, but common traits associated with autism include difficulty talking, repeated behaviors, and aversion to loud noises. ASD impedes an individual's communication skills, making it difficult to learn or to integrate socially. There are no medical treatments for autism itself; however, medications and behavioral therapy can help mitigate certain symptoms. While there is currently no known cause or cure for autism, research to determine the cause or causes may identify risk factors, some of which may be modifiable. Other studies may determine optimal methods of screening and diagnosis, identify the most effective mental and behavioral health therapies, and find the best medical treatments for individuals with ASD.

The federal government has a role in the financing (through Medicaid and State Children's Health Insurance Programs) and delivery (through funding of developmental disabilities programming in schools, Title V Maternal and Child Health funding, and other sources) of treatment for ASD.[7]

The number of cases and their appropriate diagnosis and treatment affect federal and state expenditures.[8] As such, Congress has shown interest in financing research on ASD prevalence, causes, and optimal treatment for individuals with ASD. This interest in ASD surveillance and research has been demonstrated through inclusion of autism research provisions in the Children's Health Act (CHA, P.L. 106-310) in 2000, enactment of the Combating Autism Act in 2006 (CAA, P.L. 109-416), and the recent enactment of the Combating Autism Reauthorization Act (CARA, P.L. 112-32) by the 112th Congress.

This report presents an overview of the CAA and CARA, Department of Health and Human Services (HHS) funding and activities under the CAA and CARA, other federal activities related to autism, and selected issues for Congress.

THE COMBATING AUTISM ACT (CAA)

The precursor to the CAA was the Children's Health Act of 2000 (CHA), which addressed a number of child health issues. Title I of the CHA authorized the Secretary of HHS (the Secretary) to conduct certain activities relevant to autism and developmental disabilities. It established funding for autism surveillance at CDC and established the National Center on Birth Defects and Developmental Disabilities.

Under the CHA, the National Institutes of Health (NIH) was authorized to expand and intensify its autism research efforts and to establish Centers of Excellence for autism research. The CHA also established an Autism Coordinating Committee to coordinate research within NIH, and authorized funds for HHS to establish and implement an information and education campaign for health care providers and the general public.

Enacted in 2006 and subsequently reauthorized by the Combating Autism Reauthorization Act of 2011, the CAA is intended to address growing concern about the increasing prevalence of autism spectrum disorders, and to stimulate research into possible autism causes and treatments. It authorized funding from FY2007 through FY2011 for autism research, screening, early intervention, and education. CARA reauthorized this funding through FY2014.

The CAA authorizes the Secretary to expand, intensify, and coordinate existing ASD research activities; to expand surveillance and epidemiological research; to increase awareness of ASD; and to provide access to screening and early intervention services. It authorizes expanded research activities at NIH, and created the Interagency Autism Coordinating Committee (IACC) to coordinate all federal autism research efforts (this expanded the mission of the Autism Coordinating Committee described above).

At CDC, the CAA authorizes surveillance and establishes ASD awareness programs. At the Health Resources and Services Administration (HRSA), the CAA authorizes expanded federal efforts in autism education, early detection, and intervention.

The CAA also required a report to Congress on implementation and progress four years after enactment, which was provided to Congress on January 7, 2011.[9] CARA requires a report to Congress two years after enactment.

The following sections summarize the programs and funding authorized under the CAA and subsequently reauthorized by CARA.

Surveillance and Epidemiological Research

The CAA authorizes CDC to award competitive grants for the collection, analysis, and reporting of state-level epidemiological data on ASD and other developmental disabilities. CDC must establish guidelines for reporting these data, in collaboration with other public and private entities. CDC is also required to coordinate the federal response to potential or alleged clusters of ASD or developmental disabilities (DD).

The CAA also requires CDC to award grants or cooperative agreements for the establishment of regional centers of excellence in the epidemiology of ASD and other developmental disabilities. The purpose of the centers of excellence is to collect and analyze information on the number, incidence, correlates, and causes of ASD and other DD. The centers are required to collect and report data according to the guidelines established by CDC. In addition, centers are required to develop an area of special research expertise (such as genetics, epigenetics, or environmental epidemiology), and to identify suitable cases and controls for research into potential causes or risk factors for ASD.

Autism Education, Early Detection, and Intervention

The CAA authorizes the Secretary to provide grants for projects designed to (1) increase awareness of ASD; (2) reduce barriers to screening and diagnosis; (3) promote evidence-based interventions for individuals with ASD or other developmental disabilities; (4) train health care professionals to use valid, reliable screening tools; and (5) provide early intervention if needed. The Secretary must use an interdisciplinary approach that also focuses on specific issues for children who are not receiving early diagnosis and interventions. These activities are carried out through HRSA.

The Secretary must, subject to funding, provide information and education on ASD to increase public awareness of developmental milestones; promote research into the development and validation of reliable screening tools; promote early screening of high-risk individuals; increase the number of individuals who are able to diagnose or rule out ASD; increase the number of individuals who are able to provide evidence-based interventions; and promote the use of evidence-based interventions for high-risk individuals.

The Secretary must, subject to funding, collaborate with a number of federal programs for low-income individuals to provide culturally competent information regarding ASD and developmental disabilities, in collaboration with the Department of Education and the Department of Agriculture. These programs include Head Start; Early Start; Healthy Start; programs under the Child Care and Development Block Grant Act of 1990; Medicaid, including the Early and Periodic Screening, Diagnosis, and Treatment Program (EPSDT); the State Children's Health Insurance Plan (CHIP); the Maternal and Child Health Block Grant; Individuals with Disabilities Education Act Parts B and C; and the Special Supplemental Nutrition Program for Women, Infants, and Children (WIC).

The CAA authorizes the Secretary to require states to designate a lead agency responsible for disseminating the information described above available to individuals in the state. This information may be provided through toll-free numbers, Internet websites, mailings, or other means, as determined by the governor of each state. In addition, the Secretary, through the states, must promote and assist the development and use of screening tools. The Secretaries of HHS and the Department of Education must provide for the collection, storage, coordination, and public availability of screening tools and educational materials. The CAA also authorizes the Secretary to fund grants to expand existing interdisciplinary training and leadership programs (authorized in Title V of the Social Security Act). The Secretary must also promote best practices in autism screening and diagnosis.

Centers of Excellence in Autism Research, and Research Coordination

The CAA authorizes the Secretary of HHS to expand, intensify, and coordinate ASD research activities at NIH, and to consolidate existing program activities if necessary. It directs NIH to investigate the cause, diagnosis, early detection, prevention, services, supports, intervention, and treatment of ASD.

The CAA also authorizes the Interagency Autism Coordinating Committee (IACC) at NIH to coordinate all ASD research, screening, intervention, and education efforts within HHS. Members of the IACC are appointed for a term of four years and may be reappointed once. Members must include representatives of the following: Administration for Children and Families (ACF), CDC, Centers for Medicare and Medicaid Services (CMS), HRSA, NIH, HHS Office on Disability, Substance Abuse and Mental Health Services Administration (SAMHSA), and the Department of Education. No fewer than six members, or one-third of the committee (whichever is greater) must be non-federal public members, including people with autism, parents of people with autism, and leaders of national autism organizations.

The IACC is required to meet at least twice per year in public session. It is responsible for formulating and annually updating the strategic plan for ASD research, and presenting those recommendations to the Secretary and to Congress. The IACC must also monitor all federal ASD activities, make recommendations to the Secretary and to NIH regarding changes to these activities, and make recommendations on public participation in decision making to the Secretary.

COMBATING AUTISM REAUTHORIZATION ACT (CARA)

Funding for CAA programs was authorized through FY2011; the Combating Autism Reauthorization Act (CARA), which extends funding at current levels through FY2014, was signed into law on September 30, 2011. CARA authorizes appropriations through FY2014 for CAA activities, but does not include funding or authorizations for an expansion of research and/or other services as some autism advocates had requested.[10]

FUNDING

Table 1 presents authorizations of appropriations for the provisions of the CAA and CARA. The table includes authorizations of appropriations from FY2007 through FY2014. Table 2 provides details of funding for CAA activities, as reported by HHS.[11] Full-year appropriations for FY2013 have yet to be enacted and therefore are not included in Table 2. However, the six-month FY2013 CR (P.L. 112-175, signed into law on September 28, 2012) provided funding at FY2012 levels, increased by 0.612%. As such, the funding levels for FY2013 are estimates.[12] For CAA activities, FY2012 funding totaled $237 million. Funding for FY2013 activities is estimated at $238 million, a $1 million increase.

CAA authorizations and funding are presented in two separate tables because funding for autism-related activities is not specifically limited to the authorizations shown in Table 1, and may be more or less in a given year. In addition, agencies typically do not have disease-specific budget lines. Autism-related activities may also be funded at CDC and NIH through general authorizations. The information on agency level spending in Table 2 is compiled from the Moyer Report, a report published by the HHS Office of the Assistant Secretary for Financial Resources. The Moyer Report presents information as reported by the agencies on spending for selected diseases and conditions, including autism.

Federally funded autism research not authorized under the CAA, including activities carried out by the Departments of Defense and Education, is discussed below in the section "Other Federal Activities Related to Autism Research."

Table 1. Authorizations of Appropriations in the Combating Autism Act of 2006 and the Combating Autism Reauthorization Act of 2011 Dollars in millions

	FY2007	FY2008	FY2009	FY2010	FY2011	FY2012	FY2013	FY2014
Developmental Disabilities and Surveillance Program (PHSA 399AA)	15.0	16.5	18.0	19.5	21.0	22.0	22.0	22.0
Autism Education, Early Detection, and Intervention (PHSA 399BB)	32.0	37.0	42.0	47.0	52.0	48.0	48.0	48.0
Interagency Autism Coordinating Committee, Autism Centers of Excellence (PHSA 399CC, 409C, and 404H)	100.0	114.5	129.0	143.5	158.0	161.0	161.0	161.0
Total	147.0	168.0	189.0	210.0	231.0	231.0	231.0	231.0

Source: For FY2007 through FY2011, CAA, P.L. 109-416; FY2012 through FYFY2014, CARA, P.L. 112-32.

Notes: Appropriations are authorized in Section 399EE of the PHSA.

Table 2. Funding for Activities Related to the Combating Autism Act Dollars in millions

	FY2007	FY2008	FY2009	FY2010	FY2011	FY2012	FY2013
Centers for Disease Control and Prevention	14.8	16.2	20.4	22.1	21.4	21.3	21.3
Health Resources and Services Administration[a]	0	36.4	42.0	47.9	47.7	47.1	47.1
National Institutes of Health	126.8	118.1	254.1	159.6	168.7	169.2	169.7
Total	141.6	170.7	316.5	229.6	237.8	237.6	238.1

Sources: Compiled by the Congressional Research Service from the FY2011 Moyer Material, Office of the Assistant Secretary for Financial Resources, HHS, February 2010; the FY2012 Moyer Material, Office of the Assistant Secretary for Financial Resources, HHS, March 2011, the FY2013 Moyer Material, Office of the Assistant Secretary for Financial Resources, HHS, February 2012.

a. Prior to FY2008, HRSA autism activities were funded within the Special Projects of Regional and National Significance (SPRANS) set-aside of funds from the Maternal and Child Health Block Grant, and were not provided a separate line of funding. For the FY2013 HRSA budget request for autism activities, see http://www.hrsa.gov/about/budget/budgetjustification2013.pdf.

AUTISM ACTIVITIES UNDER THE COMBATING AUTISM ACT

The activities carried out by CDC, HRSA, and NIH under the CAA are summarized below. As discussed previously, CDC focuses on surveillance and epidemiological research, NIH on basic science and research coordination, and HRSA on autism education, detection, and early intervention. For further detail on agencies' autism-related activities and publications, refer to the IACC's Report to Congress on Activities Related to Autism Spectrum Disorder and Other Developmental Disabilities Under the Combating Autism Act of 2006.[13]

Centers for Disease Control and Prevention (CDC)

Under the Combating Autism Act, the CDC is responsible for ASD and developmental disabilities surveillance and epidemiological research. Under the CHA and CAA, CDC formed the National Center on Birth Defects and Developmental Disabilities, the Autism and Developmental Disabilities Monitoring Network (ADDM), and the Centers for Autism and Developmental Disabilities Research and Epidemiology (CADDRE), an ASD education campaign for caregivers and health professionals, and has collaborated on the International Autism Epidemiology Network (IAEN).[14] CDC also coordinates with other agencies, including HRSA and the Department of the Army, on other epidemiologic ASD research.

The National Center on Birth Defects and Developmental Disabilities established the ADDM network for the collection, analysis, and reporting of state-level epidemiological data on ASD and other developmental disabilities. ADDM monitors the prevalence of ASD among eight-year-olds at selected sites. The sites, which are regional or state-based public or private nonprofit entities, collect data on ASD prevalence using uniform surveillance methods, which include screening health and education records at multiple sources. Pilot surveillance sites were established with funding from the Children's Health Act; the program was expanded to additional sites under the CAA. ADDM has published two widely cited reports on ASD prevalence, one in 2007 and another in 2009.[15]

Under the CAA, CDC established a grant program for states or other entities (e.g., private nonprofits institutions, including institutions of higher education and hospitals) to establish regional centers of excellence in ASD. These centers, called the Centers for Autism Developmental Disabilities Research and Epidemiology (CADDRE), are part of a multi-site collaborative study examining the risk factors for ASD and other developmental disabilities.[16]

The CADDRE network is currently working on the Study to Explore Early Development (SEED), which seeks to characterize ASD-related traits.[17]

CDC has partnered with the autism advocacy organization Autism Speaks to compile statistics on the global prevalence of autism. This partnership is called the International Autism Epidemiology Network.[18] The IAEN has produced a fact sheet that summarizes global autism prevalence from 2000 to 2008.[19]

In addition to research and surveillance activities, CDC has established a health communication campaign, entitled "Learn the Signs. Act Early," to improve early identification of children with ASD. The campaign is intended to educate parents, health care professionals, and early educators on the developmental milestones of early childhood.

Health Resources and Services Administration (HRSA)

Under the CAA, the Maternal and Child Health Bureau of HRSA must ensure that children with ASD are screened, diagnosed, and receive appropriate treatment. It is also tasked with addressing the shortage of trained professionals who provide autism treatment. HRSA received funding to address the five following objectives: (1) to increase awareness of ASD; (2) to reduce barriers to screening and diagnosis; (3) to promote evidence-based interventions for individuals with ASD or other developmental disabilities; (4) to train health care professionals to use valid, reliable screening tools; and (5) to provide early intervention if needed. To address these objectives, HRSA established or increased support for four programs: Leadership Education in Neurodevelopmental Disabilities (LEND), Developmental Behavioral Pediatric training programs, state implementation programs, and research programs.

HRSA has used CAA funding to support 43 LEND programs and 10 Developmental Behavioral Pediatric training programs by public and private nonprofit agencies in FY2011. The programs focus on the use of screening and diagnostic tools, and continuing education for health care providers that serve women, children, and families. These programs are designed to address the shortage of qualified professionals available to assess and assist autistic individuals.

The governor of each state must designate a lead agency to coordinate the HRSA-funded activities in that state. HRSA state-level grantees have used their funds to implement state autism plans, promote autism awareness, and develop model systems of services for children with ASD and developmental disabilities.[20] The primary focus of state implementation grants is to improve access to ASD and developmental disabilities screening and diagnostic services.

HRSA has established Autism Intervention Research programs, focusing on interventions to improve the health and well-being of children and adolescents with ASD and other developmental disabilities. These grants are provided to develop research networks among public and non-profit private institutions that focus on evidence-based research and the development of best practices in physical health, behavioral health, and the general health and well-being of individuals with ASD. Autism Intervention Research programs develop evidence-based guidelines and test and validate tools for measuring treatment outcomes.

National Institutes of Health (NIH)

CAA funding at NIH supports intramural and extramural research[21] at multiple institutes and centers. Under the CAA, NIH-funded researchers are tasked with studying potential risk factors and causes of autism, and to coordinate and consolidate its research on ASD and other developmental disabilities with other agencies.

NIH supports and coordinates the Autism Centers of Excellence Program, consisting of 11 research centers and networks that focus on identifying the causes of ASD and developing treatments. This includes research on biomarkers, genetic susceptibility, pharmacotherapy, language development, early intervention, and risk and protective factors. Another study, the Early Autism Risk Longitudinal Investigation, is looking into the interaction of environmental and genetic factors in ASD.[22]

NIH has sponsored a number of scientific workshops and symposia on ASD-related research. NIH also supports ASD research infrastructure, including biobanking (storage and archiving of biological samples) support, and the establishment of a common database (the National Database for Autism Research) to warehouse data collected in NIH-funded ASD studies.

The Children's Health Act required NIH to form a committee to coordinate research among the Institutes. The CAA broadened the mission of the coordinating committee to include other entities, both within and outside of HHS. The Interagency Autism Coordinating Committee (IACC), chaired by the director of the National Institute for Mental Health, is intended to facilitate the exchange of information on autism activities among the member agencies, and coordinates HHS autism-related programs and initiatives. The CAA required the IACC to present a strategic plan for ASD research, focusing on gaps, opportunities, and new knowledge in the autism research field. The strategic plan must be updated annually. The 2011 IACC Strategic Plan, released on February 28, 2011, includes a new focus on interventions for non-verbal people with ASD, health promotion efforts, and safety.[23]

OTHER FEDERAL ACTIVITIES RELATED TO AUTISM RESEARCH

Federal funding for autism research is not limited to the Combating Autism Act, and is supported by the Department of Defense and the Department of Education in addition to HHS. Many of the stakeholders in the IACC do not receive funding under the CAA, but through their participation in autism research, these stakeholders have an interest and a guiding role. Following is a brief description of the autism-related research activities of the other federal participants in the IACC.

Other HHS Agencies

Certain HHS agencies employ general authorities to direct funds as needed to address public health concerns. For example, CDC may provide funding for autism programs under its general authorities to fund public health activities. Other relevant activities may focus broadly on developmental disabilities and receive funding under different authorities. Within HHS, ACF, CMS, the Office on Disability, and SAMHSA conduct activities that contribute to the growing body of research on ASD. The CAA does not authorize appropriations for these agencies.

ACF is the HHS agency responsible for federal programs that promote the economic and social well-being of families, including Head Start and Temporary Assistance for Needy Families. The agency participates in the IACC and provides services for children with ASD through funds authorized under the Developmental Disabilities Assistance and Bill of Rights Act of 2000 (P.L. 106-402). ACF funds state Developmental Disabilities Councils; Protection and Advocacy Agencies; Centers for Excellence in Developmental Disabilities Education, Research, and Services; and Projects of National Significance.[24]

CMS administers the Medicare, Medicaid, and State Children's Health Insurance Program. The agency participates in the IACC and supports autism education, early detection, and intervention services under the CAA through Medicaid's EPSDT program.[25] CMS has also conducted several studies on best practices in autism treatment, and is planning to issue a report of all state services available to individuals with ASD.

The HHS Office on Disability is primarily a policy office that supports coordination of resources across HHS and federal agencies to support individuals with disabilities, including those with autism.[26]

Finally, SAMHSA is the HHS agency responsible for supporting mental health and substance abuse programs.[27] The agency provides services to children with ASD through the Child Mental Health Initiative, a grant program mandated by Congress to serve children and youth with serious emotional disorders. This program provides grants for the development of coordinated support systems for children who are referred to the program.

Non-HHS Agencies

Federal autism activities are not limited to HHS agencies. Other federal entities use general authorities and previously established programs to address ASD. These entities include the Department of Defense (DOD) and the Department of Education.

The DOD does not receive funds under the CAA. However, it maintains a congressionally directed research program for ASD research, which was first funded in FY2007.[28] The program, which supports a range of scientific and clinical research on autism, received $41 million in total funding from FY2007 to FY2012.[29]

The Department of Education does not receive appropriations under the CAA.[30] However, it funds a number of research programs and collects data on individuals served by special education programs. Programs and services in the Department of Education are geared toward individuals with disabilities in general, and not autism or developmental disabilities specifically.

Coordination of Public and Private Autism Research Funding

In 2010, the IACC conducted an analysis of autism research spending by private and federal entities that are represented on the IACC.[31] Analysts found that private entities funded 24% of autism research in the United States in 2009, while the federal government funded 76%. The report also gauged the relevance of the funded projects to the topic areas that were identified in the IACC strategic plan.[32] These objectives for 2009 were (1) When should I be concerned? (2) How can I understand what is happening? (3) What caused this to happen and can it be prevented? (4) Which treatments and interventions will help? (5) Where can I turn for services? (6) What does the future hold, particularly for adults? (7) What other infrastructure and surveillance needs must be met? The vast majority (95%) of ASD research aligned with research questions in the IACC strategic plan, with the largest proportion of research focused on the causes and prevention of ASD. Research on access to ASD-related services and lifespan issues received the least amount of funding.

ISSUES FOR CONGRESS

During CAA enactment and reauthorization, several issues were highlighted, some of which are of general interest to Congress when deciding whether to support disease-specific legislation. Specifically, concerns were raised about barriers to data sharing and confidentiality across state and federal government entities; the coordination of surveillance and research, across both agencies and diseases; and the pros and cons of Congress directing funding to specific diseases (or groups of diseases). These concerns apply not only to autism research policy, but can be applied broadly to any disease-specific legislation, and the consequent policy decisions may affect access to care and treatment for individuals with autism.

Coordination of research and sharing of the resulting data is an ongoing interest of Congress. Researchers call for accurate case estimates in order to study common characteristics of autistic individuals and potential risk factors for autism. Federal and state-funded programs provided through health care providers and schools must provide certain services for individuals with ASD, and need accurate estimates to anticipate the need for those services. However, enumerating autism cases for researchers, health care providers, and schools has presented an ongoing challenge at the state, local, and federal levels.[33]

During the reauthorization process, some Members of Congress raised the concern that continuing to pass disease-specific legislation allows Congress to prioritize one disease (or group of diseases, in this case developmental disabilities) over another, and that priority-setting should be left to the agencies that perform the research. The issue of prioritizing one developmental disability over another has also been raised among researchers and families of children with developmental disabilities and other conditions. Advocates for CARA argued that allowing authorization of these programs to lapse would interrupt the progress made under the CAA.

Autism services research, such as the development and adoption of new screening tools and implementation of best practices in autism therapy, has effects on both health care cost and coverage decisions made at the government and individual level. The Patient Protection and Affordable Care Act (ACA, P.L. 111-148) includes provisions that may affect coverage for individuals with autism, including prohibitions on the cancellation of coverage by an insurer due to a preexisting condition, elimination of lifetime caps on insurance benefits and annual limits on coverage, and eligibility for tax subsidies to assist low- and middle-income individuals in the purchase of coverage from state health insurance exchanges. In addition, Medicaid eligibility will be broadened to include single adults. The long-range impact of health reform on individuals with ASD (specifically, the coverage of recommended treatments for ASD) is unknown.

APPENDIX. LIST OF ACRONYMS

ACA	Patient Protection and Affordable Care Act, P.L. 111-148
ACF	Administration for Children and Families
ADDM	Autism and Developmental Disabilities Monitoring Network
ASD	Autism Spectrum Disorder
CAA	Combating Autism Act
CADDRE	Centers for Autism and Developmental Disabilities Research and Epidemiology
CARA	Combating Autism Reauthorization Act
CDC	Centers for Disease Control and Prevention
CHA	Children's Health Act
CHIP	State Children's Health Insurance Program
CMS	Centers for Medicare and Medicaid Services
DD	Developmental Disabilities
DOD	Department of Defense
EPSDT	Early Periodic Screening, Diagnosis, and Treatment Program
HHS	Department of Health and Human Services
HRSA	Health Resources and Services Administration
IACC	Interagency Autism Coordinating Committee
IAEN	International Autism Epidemiology Network
LEND	Leadership Education in Neurodevelopmental Disabilities
NIH	National Institutes of Health
SAMHSA	Substance Abuse and Mental Health Services Administration

WIC	State Supplemental Nutrition Program for Women, Infants, and Children

End Notes

[1] National Institute of Mental Health, *What Are Autism Spectrum Disorders?* http://www.nimh.nih.gov/health/publications/autism/what-are-the-autism-spectrum-disorders.shtml.

[2] As defined by the *Diagnostic and Statistical Manual of Mental Disorders—Fourth Edition*.

[3] A genetic marker is a DNA sequence with a known physical location on a chromosome. Genetic markers can help link an inherited disease with the responsible gene.

[4] A biologic marker is a measurable and quantifiable parameter that serves as an indicator for health and physiology assessments, such as disease risk, environmental exposures, metabolic processes, etc. For example, the presence of antibodies in a blood sample may indicate an infection.

[5] Autism and Developmental Disabilities Monitoring Network, *Prevalence of Autism Spectrum Disorders*, United States, 2006, Atlanta, GA, December 18, 2009, http://www.cdc.gov /mmwr/preview/mmwrhtml/ss5810a1.htm.

[6] National Institute of Mental Health, "Autism: The Whys of Increased Prevalence," press release, November 23, 2009, http://www.nimh.nih.gov/media/video/bearman.shtml.

[7] See CRS Report RL33202, *Medicaid: A Primer*, by Elicia J. Herz; CRS Report R40444, *State Children's Health Insurance Program (CHIP): A Brief Overview*, by Elicia J. Herz and Evelyne P. Baumrucker; CRS Report R42428, *The Maternal and Child Health Services Block Grant: Background and Funding*, by Amalia K. Corby-Edwards; and CRS Report R41833, *The Individuals with Disabilities Education Act (IDEA), Part B: Key Statutory and Regulatory Provisions*, by Ann Lordeman.

[8] Ganz M, "The Lifetime Distribution of the Incremental Societal Costs of Autism," *Arch Pediatr Adolesc Med*, vol. 161, no. 4 (April 2007), pp. 343-349.

[9] Office of Autism Research Coordination, National Institutes of Health, Report to Congress on Activities Related to Autism Spectrum Disorder and Other Developmental Disabilities Under the Combating Autism Act of 2006, U.S. Department of Health and Human Services, December 2010, http://iacc.hhs.gov/reports/reports-to-congress/FY2006- 2009/index.shtml.

[10] A number of bills addressing expansion of research, global surveillance, and services for individuals with autism were introduced in the 112th Congress.

[11] FY2013 Moyer Material, Office of the Assistant Secretary for Financial Resources, HHS, February 2012.

[12] The President's Budget Requests for CDC and HRSA for FY2013 can be found at Health Resources and Services Administration, *Justification of Estimates for Appropriations Committees*, Fiscal Year 2013, February 13, 2012, http://www.hrsa.gov/about/budget /budgetjustification2013.pdf; and Centers for Disease Control and Prevention, *Justification of Estimates for Appropriations Committees*, Fiscal Year 2013, February 13, 2012, http://www.cdc.gov/ fmo/topic/Budget%20Information/appropriations_budget_form_pdf/FY2013_CDC_CJ_Final.pdf. NIH does not have an autism-specific budget line.

[13] Office of Autism Research Coordination, National Institutes of Health, *Report to Congress on Activities Related to Autism Spectrum Disorder and Other Developmental Disabilities*

Under the Combating Autism Act of 2006, U.S. Department of Health and Human Services, December 2010, http://iacc.hhs.gov/reports/reports-to-congress/FY2006- 2009/index.shtml.

[14] See http://www.autismepidemiology.net/.

[15] Prevalence of Autism Spectrum Disorders, Autism and Developmental Disabilities Monitoring Network, Six Sites, United States, 2000, Autism and Developmental Disabilities Monitoring Network, Atlanta, GA, February 9, 2007, http://www.cdc.gov/mmwr/preview/mmwrhtml /ss5601a1.htm; Prevalence of Autism Spectrum Disorders, Autism and Developmental Disabilities Monitoring Network, United States, 2006, Autism and Developmental Disabilities Monitoring Network, Atlanta, GA, December 18, 2009, http://www.cdc.gov/mmwr/preview/mmwrhtml/ss5810a1.htm.

[16] See http://www.cdc.gov/ncbddd/autism/caddre.html.

[17] See http://www.cdc.gov/ncbddd/autism/seed.html.

[18] Centers for Disease Control and Prevention and Autism Speaks, "International Autism Epidemiology Network," press release, 2009, http://www.autismepidemiology.net/.

[19] International Autism Epidemiology Network, "Autism Prevalence Around the World (2000-2008)," press release, 2009, http://www.worldautismawarenessday.org/atf/.

[20] See http://mchb.hrsa.gov/programs/autism/statedempolicy.html.

[21] *Extramural research* is performed by non-federal scientists using NIH grant or contract money; *intramural research* is performed by NIH scientists in the NIH laboratories and Clinical Center.

[22] See http://www.earlistudy.org/.

[23] Interagency Autism Coordinating Committee, *2011 Strategic Plan for Autism Spectrum Disorder Research*, January 2011, http://www.iacc.hhs.gov/strategic-plan/2011/IACC_ 2011_Strategic_Plan.pdf.

[24] See the Administration on Developmental Disabilities, ACF: http://www.acf.hhs.gov /programs/add/.

[25] See CRS Report RL33202, *Medicaid: A Primer*, by Elicia J. Herz.

[26] See the Office on Disability: http://www.hhs.gov/od/index.html.

[27] See SAMHSA: http://www.samhsa.gov/.

[28] U.S. Congress, Senate Committee on Appropriations, *Department of Defense Appropriations Bill, 2007*, report to accompany H.R. 5631, 109th Cong., 2nd sess., July 25, 2006, 109-292 (Washington: GPO, 2006), p. 223.

[29] Congressionally Directed Medical Research Programs: http://cdmrp.army.mil/arp/default. shtml.

[30] However, individuals with autism are entitled to a free and appropriate public education under the Individuals with Disabilities Education Act (IDEA, P.L. 101-476, as amended), and public school systems provide services for children with autism from ages 6 to 21. Currently, 300,000 children with autism receive services under IDEA, and more than 6,000 individuals with autism participate in their vocational rehabilitation programs.

[31] Office of Autism Research Coordination, Interagency Autism Coordinating Committee, *2009 Autism Spectrum Disorder Research Portfolio Analysis Report*, June 2011, http://iacc.hhs.gov/portfolio-analysis/2009/ 2009_portfolio_analysis.pdf.

[32] Interagency Autism Coordinating Committee, *2011 Strategic Plan for Autism Spectrum Disorder Research*, January 2011, http://www.iacc.hhs.gov/strategic-plan/2011/IACC_ 2011_Strategic_Plan.pdf.

[33] U.S. Government Accountability Office, *Federal Autism Activities: Funding for Research has Increased, but Agencies Need to Resolve surveillance Challenges*, 06-700, July 2006, p. 12, http://www.gao.gov/new.items/ d06700.pdf.

In: The Combating Autism Act
Editor: Deryck Harlow
ISBN: 978-1-63321-128-5

Chapter 2

COMBATING AUTISM ACT: HHS AGENCIES RESPONDED WITH NEW AND CONTINUING ACTIVITIES, INCLUDING OVERSIGHT*

United States Government Accountability Office

WHY GAO DID THIS STUDY

CDC considers autism to be an important public health concern. In 2012, CDC reported that an estimated 1 in 88 children in the United States has been identified as having autism— a 23 percent increase from its estimate of 1 in 110 reported in 2009. Autism is a developmental disorder involving communication and social impairment. Symptoms usually become evident in early childhood. There are many suspected causes and no known cure.

HHS agencies fund educational and support services for individuals diagnosed with autism and fund research in a variety of areas, such as identifying the causes of autism and intervention options. The CAA amended sections of the Children's Health Act of 2000 related to autism and established new requirements. The CAA, enacted in December 2006, authorized the expansion of HHS's activities related to autism research, surveillance, prevention, intervention, and education through fiscal year 2011. The CAA

* This is an edited, reformatted and augmented version of United States Government Accountability Office Publication, No. GAO-13-232, dated February 2013.

authorized, but did not appropriate, federal funding to carry out these activities.

In this report, GAO (1) describes the actions that HHS agencies have taken as a result of the CAA, and (2) examines the oversight of CAA grantees. To address these objectives, GAO reviewed CAA and HHS documents and interviewed agency officials to identify the autism activities resulting from the CAA. GAO also determined the amount certain HHS agencies spent on autism activities from fiscal year 2006—prior to the CAA—through fiscal year 2011. In addition, GAO reviewed files for a random sample of CAA grantees to examine oversight from 2008 to 2011.

WHAT GAO FOUND

Department of Health and Human Services (HHS) agencies responded to the Combating Autism Act of 2006 (CAA) by establishing some new autism activities and continuing others. The Health Resources and Services Administration (HRSA) created a new initiative to address specific directives in the CAA. Through this initiative, HRSA expanded its existing training programs by requiring grantees to include training specific to autism. It also established new autism research grants and funded new state grants to improve services for children with autism. HRSA awards its autism grants under the authority of the CAA. The National Institutes of Health (NIH) and Centers for Disease Control and Prevention (CDC) continued their autism activities—some of which were undertaken in response to the Children's Health Act of 2000—but did not create new programs as a direct result of the CAA. NIH continued to fund, expand, and coordinate autism research through its Autism Centers of Excellence and autism-specific grants and contracts. CDC continued to fund its regional centers of excellence for autism epidemiology and other activities, such as an awareness campaign. HHS's Interagency Autism Coordinating Committee (IACC)— reauthorized by the CAA—assumed additional responsibilities to coordinate autism efforts within HHS and restructured its membership to include more nonfederal members. NIH created the Office of Autism Research Coordination to coordinate and manage the IACC. The CAA did not appropriate funds to any HHS agency. Nevertheless, overall spending on HRSA, NIH, CDC, and IACC autism activities increased from approximately $143.6 million in fiscal year 2006 to approximately $240.4 million in fiscal year 2011.

HRSA, the only HHS agency that has awarded grants specifically as a result of the CAA, regularly collects and reviews information from grantees to oversee individual CAA grantees and programs. HRSA awarded approximately $164 million in grants to 110 CAA grantees from fiscal years 2008 to 2011; though, some of these grantees were already receiving funds prior to the CAA. To oversee these grantees, HRSA requires they regularly submit progress reports and financial reports. The agency also requires grantees to obtain prior approval before making certain changes to their projects. GAO reviewed documentation for an unbiased random sample of 22 grantees, which were representative of the 110 CAA grantees. GAO found that CAA grantees submitted all required reports. Many grantees submitted prior-approval requests for changes to their projects. Most frequently, grantees requested to carry over unobligated funds from the current year to the next budget period. GAO found that HRSA staff routinely collected and reviewed information submitted by the grantees and appropriately documented their review and approval of these submissions. HRSA also conducted site visits and provided technical assistance as a means of overseeing grantees. HRSA conducted site visits with 9 of the grantees in our sample during the period of our review, while only 2 of these were required sites visits. Besides overseeing grantees, HRSA monitors its overall CAA programs by regularly collecting performance reports from grantees. In addition, in December 2012, HRSA released a grant-management operations manual to outline its overall approach for monitoring its CAA programs.

GAO provided a draft of this report to HHS for comment. In response, HHS provided technical comments that were incorporated, as appropriate.

ABBREVIATIONS

CAA	Combating Autism Act of 2006
CDC	Centers for Disease Control and Prevention
DBP	Developmental-Behavioral Pediatrics
EHB	Electronic Handbook
HHS	Department of Health and Human Services
HRSA	Health Resources and Services Administration
IACC	Interagency Autism Coordinating Committee
LEND	Leadership Education in Neurodevelopmental and Other Related Disabilities
NIH	National Institutes of Health

NIMH	National Institute of Mental Health
OARC	Office of Autism Research Coordination

February 27, 2013

Congressional Requesters

The Centers for Disease Control and Prevention (CDC) considers autism to be an important public health concern. In March 2012, CDC—an agency within the Department of Health and Human Services (HHS)— reported that an estimated 1 in 88 children in the United States had been identified as having autism—a 23 percent increase from its estimate of 1 in 110 children in 2009.[1] Autism is characterized by impaired social interactions, problems with verbal and nonverbal communication, and repetitive behaviors, or by severely limited activities and interests. What is commonly known as "autism" is a group of disorders known as autism spectrum disorders.[2] Diagnoses include autistic disorder, a more severe form of autism, and Asperger syndrome, a milder form of autism.

HHS agencies fund educational and support services for individuals diagnosed with autism and fund research, such as studies to identify the causes of autism and intervention options. Some of HHS's autism-related activities are performed internally by its agencies, while others are conducted by external organizations. For example, HHS agencies award grants to institutions to conduct autism-related research and surveillance activities. Each HHS agency is responsible for overseeing the funds that it awards to external organizations to ensure that they are properly and effectively used.

To address growing concern about the increasing prevalence of autism and to stimulate research into possible autism causes and interventions, the Combating Autism Act of 2006 (CAA) was enacted in December 2006.[3] The CAA authorizes the expansion of HHS's activities related to autism research, surveillance, prevention, intervention, and education and authorizes funding for such activities through fiscal year 2011.[4] You asked us to provide information on agencies' responses to the CAA and oversight of CAA activities. In this report, we (1) describe the actions that HHS agencies have taken as a result of the CAA, and (2) examine the oversight of CAA grantees.[5]

To describe the actions HHS agencies have taken as a result of the CAA, we reviewed CAA and agency documents and interviewed HHS officials. We focused our work on those HHS agencies directed to conduct autism activities included in the CAA—the Health Resources and Services Administration (HRSA), the National Institutes of Health (NIH), and CDC.[6] We reviewed documents and interviewed agency officials to identify the autism activities each agency funded, whether those activities resulted from the CAA, and the amount spent on those activities. We included activities in our review that the agencies funded from fiscal years 2006 through 2011. Although the CAA was enacted during fiscal year 2007, we included fiscal year 2006 in our analysis to help determine the extent to which these agencies' activities and funding for autism activities changed following the enactment of the CAA.

To examine the oversight of CAA grantees, we interviewed HHS officials at HRSA, NIH, and CDC to determine whether they had awarded CAA grants; reviewed agencies' grants oversight policies and procedures; and conducted a review of selected grantees' files. Specifically, we reviewed agency guidance documents that outline protocols and procedures for overseeing grantees. [7] We also reviewed documents—such as funding opportunity announcements for CAA grants—that outline CAA grantees' specific reporting requirements and other responsibilities. In addition, we interviewed agency officials about (1) policies and procedures for overseeing grantees and required oversight documentation, (2) the roles and responsibilities of various agency staff in the oversight process, and (3) grantee requirements. Lastly, we compared the grantee monitoring processes described by agency officials and documents to actual oversight activities.

To do this, we selected an unbiased random sample of 20 percent of the CAA grantees—22 of the 110—funded between 2008 and 2011 and examined grant files and related documents.[8] Our file review of the selected grantees included a review of required reports and requests grantees submitted; oversight of such reports and requests; and other documentation, such as site visit summaries, for the grants awarded in fiscal years 2008 through 2011. We reviewed documentation located in two data systems—the Electronic Handbook (EHB) and the Discretionary Grant Information System—that, according to agency officials, contain all significant documentation related to monitoring CAA grantees.[9]

To conduct this file review, we developed and used a data-collection instrument to assess whether the files included evidence of required monitoring and key monitoring documents. For example, we reviewed whether grantees submitted required reports on time, and if agency officials appropriately documented their review and approval of these reports. While we identified key monitoring actions and documents, we did not assess the quality of these actions or documents.

To assess the reliability of the data collected, we compared the information contained in the oversight documents we reviewed, information provided to us by agency officials, and information contained in the two data systems. If there were discrepancies between these sources of information, we asked HRSA to resolve the discrepancies and provide associated documentation. We found the data reliable for our purposes.

We conducted this performance audit from March 2012 to February 2013 in accordance with generally accepted government auditing standards. Those standards require that we plan and perform the audit to obtain sufficient, appropriate evidence to provide a reasonable basis for our findings based on our audit objectives. We believe that the evidence obtained provides a reasonable basis for our findings and conclusions based on our audit objectives.

BACKGROUND

Autism—a complex and pervasive developmental disability—usually becomes evident in early childhood, although signs and symptoms vary.[10] According to CDC, autism begins before age 3 and lasts throughout a person's life. Some children show signs of autism within the first few months of life. In others, symptoms might not appear until 24 months or later. Still other children with autism seem to develop typically until 18 to 24 months of age and then stop gaining new skills or lose the skills they once had. Signs and symptoms of autism include a child not responding to his or her name by 12 months; not pointing at objects to show interest by 14 months; avoiding eye contact and wanting to be alone; repeating words or phrases over and over; and flapping hands, rocking, or spinning in circles. Individuals with autism might have challenges with showing or talking about their feelings and might also have trouble understanding the feelings of others.

Diagnosing autism can be difficult; however, early intervention services can greatly improve a child's development. There is no medical diagnostic test available for autism. As a result, doctors consider a child's behavior and development to make a clinical diagnosis. By age 2, a diagnosis by an experienced professional can be considered very reliable. However, according to CDC most children do not receive a diagnosis until after age 4. There is no single cause of autism, but a variety of factors are suspected of causing or contributing to autism, including environmental, biological, and genetic sources. While there is no known cure, research shows that early intervention services can greatly improve a child's development. Because of the complexity of this disorder, individuals with autism have diverse needs for medical and mental health care as well as an array of educational and social services.

The CAA authorizes and directs HHS to conduct specific autism-related activities, which may include funding external organizations to conduct these activities through grants, contracts, and cooperative agreements.[11] The CAA amended sections of the Children's Health Act of 2000—which required HHS to conduct activities related to autism research, surveillance, and coordination—by revising some sections and repealing other sections of that law as well as establishing new requirements.[12]

The CAA authorized, but did not appropriate, federal funding to carry out these activities in fiscal year 2007 through fiscal year 2011.

HHS Agencies Responded to the CAA by Establishing New Autism Activities and Continuing Others

HHS agencies responded to the CAA with new or continuing autism activities. In fiscal year 2008, HRSA created the *Combating Autism Act Initiative* in response to specific directives included in the CAA.[13] Through this initiative, HRSA expanded its existing training programs to include an autism-specific component and established new autism research and state grants. HRSA conducts all of its *Combating Autism Act Initiative* programs under the authority of the CAA.

HRSA staff told us that they have not analyzed whether the agency's new programs could be conducted under other HRSA authority.

HRSA expanded two of its preexisting training programs—the Leadership Education in Neurodevelopmental and Other Related Disabilities (LEND) and the Developmental-Behavioral Pediatrics (DBP) training programs— through supplemental funding to existing grantees and awards to new grantees. These two training programs account for the majority of HRSA spending under its *Combating Autism Act Initiative*; however, HRSA was funding these programs prior to enactment of the CAA. 14 Under the *Combating Autism Act Initiative*, LEND and DBP grantees are required to include an autism component in their training.

Among other things, the programs train health care professionals, such as pediatric practitioners, residents, and graduate students, to provide evidence-based services to children with autism and other developmental disabilities and their families; and train specialists to provide comprehensive diagnostic evaluations to address the shortage of professionals who can confirm or rule out an autism diagnosis. According to HRSA, as a result of these training programs, the number of health professionals enrolled in autism courses increased from 1,887 in academic year 2008-2009 to 4,256 in academic year 2010-2011 and the number of diagnostic evaluations increased from 12,390 in academic year 2008-2009 to 44,102 in academic year 2010-2011.

Additionally, HRSA created new autism research programs to fund studies that are intended to advance the current autism knowledge base and lead to improvements in interventions that address the health and well-being of children and adolescents with autism and other developmental disabilities. HRSA also provided grants to establish two research networks that focus on the physical and behavioral health needs of children and adolescents with autism. These networks conduct research on evidence-based practices for interventions, promote the development of evidence-based guidelines for intervention, validate tools for autism intervention, and disseminate information to health professionals and the public, especially families affected by autism.

HRSA also funded new state implementation and planning grants to implement plans to improve access to comprehensive, coordinated health care and related services for children and youth with autism and other developmental disabilities.

Twenty-two states received grants from fiscal years 2008 to 2011 to implement their autism plans.[15] These plans vary by state, but common elements include a focus on partnerships between professionals and families of children and youth with autism, access to a culturally competent family-centered medical home, access to adequate health insurance and financing of services, early and continuous screening for autism and other developmental disabilities, community services organized for easy use by families, and transition services for youth entering adult health care. Table 1 provides information on the specific autism-related programs HRSA initiated or expanded—by increasing funding and the number of grantees—as a result of the CAA.

Table 1. Autism Programs and Funding Sponsored by the Health Resources and Services Administration (HRSA) as a Result of the Combating Autism Act, Fiscal Years 2008-2011

Programs	Type of program	Purpose of program	Number of grantees, fiscal years 2008-2011	Total funding, fiscalyears 2008-2011(dollars in millions)
Leadership Education in Neurodevelopmental and Other Related Disabilities (LEND) Training Program	Training	Improve the health of children who have, or are at risk for developing, neurodevelopmental and other related disabilities by training professionals to assume leadership roles, and to ensure high levels of interdisciplinary clinical competence in an effort to increase diagnosis of or rule out individuals with developmental disabilities, including autism.	47[a]	$107.2[a]
Developmental-Behavioral Pediatrics (DBP) Training Program	Training	Train the next generation of leaders in developmental-behavioral pediatrics; and provide pediatric practitioners, residents, and medical students with essential biopsychosocial knowledge and clinical expertise. This program is focused on developmental disabilities, including autism.	10	7.3
National Combating Autism Interdisciplinary Training Resource Center	Training	Improve the health of children who have, or are at risk for developing, autism and other developmental disabilities by providing technical assistance to LEND and DBP programs to better train professionals to utilize valid and reliable screening tools for diagnosing or ruling out autism, and provide evidence-based interventions for children.	1	2.5

Table 1. (Continued)

Programs	Type of program	Purpose of program	Number of grantees, fiscal years 2008-2011	Total funding, fiscalyears 2008-2011(dollars in millions)
Autism Intervention Research Program and Autism Intervention Secondary Data Analysis Studies Program	Research	Support research on evidence-based practices for interventions to improve the health and well-being of children and adolescents with autism and other developmental disabilities. The Autism Intervention Secondary Data Analysis Studies Program utilizes the analysis of existing secondary data.	26b	10.0b
Autism Intervention Research Network on Physical Health	Research	Establish and maintain a network infrastructure designed to be the platform from which to conduct research on evidence-based practices for interventions to improve the physical health and well-being of individuals with autism and other developmental disabilities; develop evidence-based guidelines and validate tools for interventions; and disseminate critical information on its research findings, guidelines, and tools.	1	15.6
Autism Intervention Research Network on Behavioral Health	Research	Establish and maintain a network infrastructure designed to be the platform from which to conduct research on evidence-based interventions to improve the behavioral, mental, social, or cognitive health, or a mix of those, and well-being of children and adolescents with autism and other developmental disabilities; develop evidence-based guidelines and validate tools for interventions;	1	7.9

Programs	Type of program	Purpose of program	Number of grantees, fiscal years 2008-2011	Total funding, fiscalyears 2008-2011(dollars in millions)
		and disseminate critical information on its research findings, guidelines, and tools.		
Developmental-Behavioral Pediatric Research Network	Research	Establish a multicenter scientific and clinical research network that will promote coordinated research activities and address health issues. Build a developmental behavioral pediatric research infrastructure that supports multidisciplinary research, focuses on the translation of research to practice, and provides the environment in which to train a new generation of developmental behavioral pediatric researchers.	1	0.4
State Implementation and Planning Grantsc	Other	Improve access to comprehensive, coordinated health care and related services by implementing state plans to improve the system of services.	22	11.8d
State Public Health Coordinating Center	Other	Improve the health of children who have, or are at risk for developing, autism and other developmental disabilities by coordinating with the state implementation and planning grantees; and by developing a strategy for defining, supporting, and monitoring the role of state public health agencies in assuring early and timely identification, diagnosis, and intervention.	1	1.1
Total			110	$163.8e

Source: GAO analysis of HRSA documents and interviews with HRSA officials.

Notes: HRSA's funds shown in this table were not appropriated by the Combating Autism Act (CAA). To fund these programs, HRSA used funds appropriated to the agency annually through the budget and appropriations process for the purpose of carrying out a variety of programs. Although the LEND and DBP training programs were established prior to the act, HRSA expanded these programs as a result of the act.

[a]These totals include one funding supplement to an existing cooperative agreement to provide technical assistance to LEND grantees. A cooperative agreement is an alternative assistance instrument used instead of a grant whenever substantial federal involvement with the recipient during performance is anticipated.

[b]These totals include one funding supplement to an existing cooperative agreement to examine current knowledge, research gaps, and methodological challenges about the life-course trajectory of individuals with autism, and develop a life-course-focused autism research agenda.

[c]This program comprises: State Implementation Grants for Improving Services for Children and Youth with Autism Spectrum Disorder and other Developmental Disabilities, and State Planning Grants for Improving Services for Children and Youth with Autism Spectrum Disorder and other Developmental Disabilities.

[d]This total includes supplemental funding provided to four state implementation and planning grantees to expand implementation of the Centers for Disease Control and Prevention's (CDC) *Learn the Signs. Act Early.* campaign, through an interagency agreement between HRSA and CDC.

[e]Individual funding entries do not sum to total due to rounding.

NIH and CDC continued the autism activities each implemented prior to the enactment of the CAA, but did not create new programs as a direct result of the CAA. Some of these activities had been undertaken in response to the Children's Health Act of 2000, which, like the CAA, charges NIH with expanding, intensifying, and coordinating research on autism. In addition, under both laws, CDC is required to conduct activities related to establishing regional centers of excellence to collect and analyze certain information on autism.[16]

Since the enactment of the CAA, NIH continued to fund, expand, and coordinate autism research through its Autism Centers of Excellence and autism-specific grants and contracts. According to agency officials, NIH awards these grants and contracts under its general Public Health Service Act authorities and not under the specific authorities provided in the CAA.[17] CDC continued to fund its regional centers of excellence for autism epidemiology and other activities, such as an awareness campaign on autism and other developmental disabilities. While enactment of the CAA did not result in any change to CDC's autism activities, CDC officials stated that the CAA provided additional focus on these efforts.

According to CDC officials, the CAA's enactment also strengthened the agency's *Learn the Signs. Act Early.* awareness campaign by elevating the importance of increasing awareness of developmental milestones to national visibility. See appendix I for a list of NIH's and CDC's autism efforts.

As required by the CAA, the Interagency Autism Coordinating Committee (IACC)—initially established under the Children's Health Act— restructured its membership and assumed additional responsibilities to coordinate autism efforts within HHS.

The CAA reauthorized the IACC and specified that the IACC include both federal and nonfederal members.[18] IACC membership expanded to include 11 nonfederal members that represented individuals with autism and parents of children with autism. In addition, it included members of the autism advocacy, research, and service-provider communities in accordance with the CAA's membership requirements.

The CAA also directed the IACC to develop and annually update a strategic plan and summary of advances in autism research, and monitor federal autism activities.[19] Since fiscal year 2007, the IACC issued several reports as a means to coordinate HHS autism efforts and monitor federal autism activities, some of which were specifically required by the CAA, such as the development of an autism strategic plan and a summary of advances in autism research.[20] See appendix II for a description of the documents produced by the IACC.

In addition to the changes to the IACC, in 2008, NIH created the Office of Autism Research Coordination (OARC) within the National Institute of Mental Health (NIMH) to coordinate and manage the IACC and related cross-agency activities, programs, and policies. OARC assists the IACC by conducting analyses and preparing reports for the IACC, assisting with the IACC's strategic planning and autism research monitoring, and providing logistical support for IACC meetings. It also supports communications through the IACC website and press releases, and responds to inquiries from the public and other government agencies.[21]

OARC officials told us that although HHS could establish an advisory committee similar to the IACC under other authority, the CAA has provided the IACC with greater visibility and increased involvement of the public and federal agencies, through, for example, the annual update of the IACC's autism strategic plan.

Following the enactment of the CAA, HHS agencies continued to fund existing activities and funded new activities. [22] Overall, spending on HRSA, NIH, CDC, and IACC autism activities increased from approximately $143.6 million in fiscal year 2006 to approximately $240.4 million in fiscal year 2011. HRSA spent more money on its autism programs beginning in fiscal year 2008 as a result of implementing its *Combating Autism Act Initiative*. From fiscal year 2008 through fiscal year 2010 HRSA increased this spending by an average of $5.75 million annually. HRSA's spending on autism programs totaled approximately $47.9 million in fiscal year 2010. In fiscal year 2011, HRSA spent slightly less on these programs.[23]

Although the CAA did not provide appropriations for NIH's and CDC's autism activities, nor did Congress provide the agencies a specific autism appropriation after the CAA's enactment, NIH and CDC increased their overall spending on autism from fiscal year 2006 to fiscal year 2011. NIH spent more money on its autism activities in fiscal years 2009 and 2010 as a result of an appropriation for scientific research that it received under the American Recovery and Reinvestment Act of 2009. And, according to CDC officials, the agency redirected a portion of its funding for infant health activities to support pilot projects implementing the agency's awareness campaign on autism and other developmental disabilities.

The IACC's funding increased significantly from fiscal year 2006 to 2011. From fiscal year 2008 through fiscal year 2011, as directed by Congress in the annual HHS appropriations act, the Secretary of Health and Human Services transferred funds to NIMH for the IACC. From fiscal year 2006 through fiscal year 2011, the IACC also received funds from the annual NIH appropriation. See appendix III for information on the funding for these agencies' and the IACC's autism-related activities.

HRSA ROUTINELY COLLECTS AND REVIEWS INFORMATION TO OVERSEE CAA GRANTEES

HRSA, the only HHS agency that awarded grants specifically as a result of the CAA, regularly collects and reviews information from grantees to oversee individual CAA grantees as well as to provide oversight to its CAA programs.[24] HRSA awarded approximately $164 million in grants to 110 CAA grantees from fiscal years 2008 to 2011.

The majority of funding—about $107 million—was awarded to 47 grantees within HRSA's LEND training program, some of which were already receiving funds prior to the CAA. In addition, nearly $24 million was awarded to two grantees to support HRSA's two autism intervention research networks. For all grantees, the amount of the grant award per year ranged widely from about $36,000 to $4 million depending on the CAA program, as shown in appendix IV.

As part of the agency's oversight of its CAA grantees, HRSA requires periodic reports from these grantees, which are reviewed by HRSA staff. HRSA project officers within the Maternal and Child Health Bureau—the bureau that administers the CAA programs—are responsible for working with CAA grantees in overseeing the programmatic and technical aspects of the grant. HRSA grants management specialists and their supervisors—grants management officers—oversee compliance with financial reporting requirements and agency grant policies and regulations. The required reports that are reviewed by HRSA staff include the following:

- **Annual federal financial report**. The annual federal financial report is an accounting of expenditures under the project in the budget period—the period for which HRSA has awarded funds to the grantee—and cumulatively for the project period.[25] The report is due after the end of the budget year.
- **Annual progress reports**. The annual progress report is part of a grantee's noncompeting continuing application and describes

grantees' progress on their grant objectives. Progress reports are due before the end of the budget period because HRSA staff use these reports to assess progress and, except for final progress reports, to determine whether to provide funding for the budget period subsequent to that covered by the report.[26]

- **Mid-project progress reports**. Mid-project progress reports provide information on grantees' progress on research objectives. These reports are required of certain research grantees and are due midway through the project period.[27]
- **Semiannual progress reports**. Semiannual progress reports include information on the grantees' most significant achievements and problems encountered during the reporting period as well as the grantees' progress on established objectives. These reports are required of research network grantees and are due midway through each budget period.[28]

In addition to reports, HRSA also requires grantees to submit written requests before making certain changes to the grant project, known as prior-approval requests. For example, a change in the director of the grant project requires prior approval, as does a request to carry over unobligated funds to the next budget period or a request for a no-cost extension—an extension for a limited period beyond the end of the project period so that the grantee can complete project activities.

When reviewing these reports and grantee prior-approval requests, HRSA staff are required to fill out checklists in the EHB in which they indicate their review and approval of the report or request.[29] The content of the review checklists varies by the type of report or request being reviewed. For example, among other questions, a progress report checklist asks if the report reflects the program's goals.

The federal financial report checklist asks HRSA staff to compare the report with data in HRSA's payment management system.[30] All review checklists include a question where HRSA staff can indicate if they have identified any issues or concerns with the report or request. In addition, when reviewing grantee information, HRSA staff may request that a report be revised with additional or corrected information.

Our review found that HRSA routinely collects and reviews information submitted by CAA grantees. Generally, grantees submitted required reports and HRSA staff documented their review of these reports. Specifically, the 22 grantees in our unbiased random sample 31 submitted all of the 106 reports they were required to submit and most of these reports were submitted on time.[32]

We found that HRSA staff filled out checklists approving all of the reports submitted or required report revisions. In many cases, HRSA staff filled out a checkbox indicating a "yes," "no," or "n/a" response to the questions. However, we noted that there were some cases where staff provided a narrative description to support their response to the question, such as a description of how the grantee is meeting the program's goals—a question in the progress report checklist. HRSA officials stated that staff are required to answer the questions in the checklist, but they are not required to provide a narrative supporting their answers.

We observed that there were few instances of HRSA staff either documenting a concern or asking for a report revision before approving the report. We encountered seven instances where a project officer approved a report, but documented a concern in a checklist. In all these instances, the project officer provided narrative describing the concern. 33 For example, in one instance, the project officer wrote that the grantee's recruitment of study subjects—parents of children with autism or other developmental disabilities—was slow. However, the project officer also stated that the grantee modified its enrollment process, which seemed to be having some positive effect and that the project officer and grantee were working together to monitor enrollment. We also identified another seven instances where HRSA staff asked for a report to be revised either with additional or corrected information. In almost all instances, the grantees submitted a revised report and HRSA staff completed a checklist indicating approval of the revised report.[34]

We also found that grantees submit a number of prior-approval requests, which HRSA staff review and generally approve. Most frequently, grantees request to carry over unobligated funds from the current year to the next budget period. For example, 13 of the 22 grantees in our review requested to carry over unobligated balances at least once during the period of our review, and many of them requested it for multiple years— equaling 32 separate requests. The amount of unobligated balances that grantees requested to carry over in a given year ranged from $1,518 to $172,514. In all instances, HRSA approved these requests as indicated by the issuance of a revised notice of award.[35] Almost all requests related to awards in fiscal year 2010 and later contained an associated checklist in the EHB filled out by HRSA staff approving the request to carry over unobligated balances.[36]

In addition to reviewing information submitted by grantees, HRSA provides additional oversight to grantees. First, it conducts site visits in person or by means of the web. During a site visit, HRSA staff may collect information on preliminary research findings, data and analysis, and any challenges the grantee is facing. Site visits are only required of certain research grantees, although HRSA may conduct site visits with other grantees, depending on available resources.[37] HRSA officials target site visits for CAA grantees on the basis of six criteria: (1) the grantee is new, (2) there has been a change in the grantee's project director, (3) there has been a change in the grantee's scope of work, (4) there are budgetary issues or the grantee has not made adequate progress on the project goals, (5) the grantee has requested technical assistance, or (6) there has been a change in the project officer overseeing the grantee. HRSA uses a site-visit report to document the visit and has guidance on what should be included in the report. For example, for training grants, the report should include a narrative summary of the visit including highlights, performance measure progress, strengths and challenges, and any technical assistance needed by the grantee. Second, HRSA officials stated that HRSA project officers provide routine technical assistance to certain grantees and others on an as-needed basis. For example, all research grantees have either a monthly, biweekly, or mid-project telephone call with HRSA project officers.

Our review confirmed that HRSA has conducted a number of site visits to monitor CAA grantees. For example, nine of the grantees in our review had documentation indicating that a site visit had been conducted, with only two of these being required site visits. While none of the site-visit reports identified major issues that required corrective action, some did record challenges the grantees were facing or made suggestions. For example, one report stated that the grantee may encounter challenges in the recruitment of trainees. We identified documentation related to technical assistance that HRSA staff provided to some grantees but not all. For example, we did not always see documentation of routine telephone calls with research grantees that HRSA officials say occur on a regular basis. In response, HRSA officials stated that not all technical assistance is recorded in the EHB; only when a significant issue arises is the telephone call, e-mail, or other assistance recorded.

Besides overseeing specific grantees, HRSA monitors its CAA activities at the program level by regularly collecting performance reports from grantees.[38] The 22 CAA grantees in our sample submitted all the required performance reports. According to HRSA officials, the primary purpose of performance reports is to gauge program performance.

For example, data in performance reports is currently being used by a HRSA contractor to prepare a report on the progress of the CAA programs for Congress.[39] In addition, according to HRSA officials, performance data can be used to modify program performance measures over time. While performance reports are used to monitor CAA programs—as opposed to grantees—HRSA officials stated that some performance information is also included in annual progress reports, which are used to oversee specific grantees. For example, progress reports require grantees to include information on whether they are having problems meeting their performance measures.

Finally, to further help oversee CAA programs and consolidate information on its monitoring approach for these programs, in December 2012 HRSA released a grant-management operations manual to outline its overall approach for monitoring these programs.[40] According to HRSA officials, this manual will be included in the program folder of the EHB for each of its CAA programs and will be reviewed annually, consistent with HHS guidance.[41]

Agency Comments

We provided a draft of this report to HHS for comment. HHS provided technical comments that we incorporated, as appropriate.

Marcia Crosse
Director, Health Care

Appendix I: National Institutes of Health's (NIH) and Centers for Disease Control and Prevention's (CDC) Autism Activities

During fiscal year 2006 through fiscal year 2011, NIH and CDC funded a number of autism activities. Table 2 lists the activities these agencies funded, including the type and purpose of each activity.

Table 2. NIH's and CDC's Autism Activities during Fiscal Years 2006 through 2011

Agency	Activity	Type of activity	Purpose of activity
NIH	Autism Centers of Excellence Program[a]	Research	NIH initiative that supports large-scale multidisciplinary studies on autism, with the goal of determining the disorders' causes and the best treatments for them.
	Collaborative Programs of Excellence in Autism[a]	Research	Conduct research to learn about the possible causes of autism, including genetic, immunological, and environmental factors; as well as diagnosis, early detection, behavioral and communications characteristics, and treatment of autism.
	Studies to Advance Autism Research and Treatment Network[a]	Research	Support and conduct both individual and collaborative projects to learn more about the causes, diagnosis, earlydetection, prevention, and treatments of autism.
	Children's Environmental Health and Disease Prevention Research Centers (with Environmental Protection Agency)[b]	Research	Examine the effect of environmental exposures on children's health.
	Research Units on Pediatric Psychopharmacology Autism Network	Research	Clinical trials evaluating psychopharmacological treatments for co-occurring behavior disorders in autism.
	Research to Address the Heterogeneity in Autism Spectrum Disorders	Research	Address gaps identified in the Interagency Autism Coordinating Committee's Strategic Plan and other knowledge gap areas related to autism, and to ensure appropriate attention is given to the most critical short-term objectives within the Strategic Plan. Applications forresearch projects were solicited within the following topicareas [relevant to research on the heterogeneity of autism]: measurement development, biomarkers/biological signatures, immune and central

Agency	Activity	Type of activity	Purpose of activity
			nervous systems interactions, genetics/genomics, environmental risk factors, model development, treatment and intervention, and services research.
	Challenge Grants in Health and Science Research[b]	Research	Support research on topic areas that address specific scientific and health research challenges in biomedical and behavioral research that would benefit from significant 2-year startup funds.
	Grand Opportunities grants[b]	Research	Support high-impact ideas that lend themselves to short-term funding, and may lay the foundation for new fields of investigation. The grants program will support large-scale research projects that accelerate critical breakthroughs, early and applied research on cutting-edge technologies, and new approaches to improve the synergy and interactions among multi- and interdisciplinary research teams. The initiative seeks novel approaches in areas that address specific knowledge gaps, scientific opportunities, new technologies, data generation, or research methods that would benefit from an influx of funds to quickly advance the area in significant ways.
	Initiative related to nonverbal school-age children	Research	Opportunity for investigators and U.S. institutions/organizations with certain active grants to submit revision applications to support an expansion of the scope or research protocol to develop preliminary investigations into the characterization and/or treatment of nonverbal school-aged children with autism.
	Contract related to Health Outcomes for Children with Autism and their Families	Research	Describe the health and health care trajectories of individuals with autism and their families, and evaluate the feasibility of using a large population-based databasefor research on risk factors for autism.
	National Institute of Mental Health Intramural Research Program, Autism Research	Research	Accelerate development and testing of innovative treatments. NIH has undertaken activities to address the effectiveness and outcomes of innovative and newly developed intervention strategies for individuals

Table 2. (Continued)

Agency	Activity	Type of activity	Purpose of activity
			diagnosed with autism or other developmental disabilities.
	Eunice Kennedy Shriver National Institute of Child Health and Human Development Brain and Tissue Bank for Developmental Disorders[b]	Research	Advance the research of developmental disorders. The objective of this human-tissue repository is to systematically collect, store, and distribute brain and other tissues for research dedicated to the improved understanding, care, and treatment of individuals with developmental disorders.
	NIH National Database for Autism Research	Research	Accelerate autism research by creating an infrastructure that integrates heterogeneous datasets allowing access to much more quality research data than investigators would be able to collect on their own.
	National Institute of Mental Health Center for Collaborative Genetic Studies of Mental Disorders[b]	Research	Accelerate progress toward understanding genetic origins of mental disorders including autism, schizophrenia, bipolar disorder, and depression. Encourage the sharing of biological as well as clinical and genetic data from individuals or families with these disorders, and perform and disseminate analyses of these data.
	Psychosocial/Behavioral Interventions and Services Research in Autism Spectrum Disorders	Research	Facilitate exploratory research on psychosocial/behavioral treatments and innovative services research for autism, including the development of instruments to evaluate the impact of interventions on core features of autism, and comorbid symptomatology.
	Research on Autism and Autism Spectrum Disorders	Research	Supports research designed to elucidate the etiology, epidemiology, diagnosis, treatment, and optimal means of service delivery in relation to autism.
	Shared Neurobiology of Fragile X Syndrome and Autism	Research	Aimed at characterizing, understanding, and treating etiological and pathophysiological mechanisms common to both Fragile X syndrome and autism.

Agency	Activity	Type of activity	Purpose of activity
	Minnesota Somali Project (with CDC)c	Surveillance	Investigate reports of elevated prevalence of autism among children born to Somali immigrants living in Minneapolis, Minn.
CDC	Metropolitan Atlanta Developmental Disabilities Surveillance Program	Surveillance	Provide regular and systematic monitoring of prevalence rates of selected developmental disabilities according to various demographic characteristics of children and theirmothers and provide a framework for initiating special studies of children who have the selected developmentaldisabilities by establishing a population-based case series of such children.
	Autism and Developmental Disabilities Monitoring Network	Surveillance	Collaborative project to characterize the population prevalence and characteristics of children with autism and other developmental disabilities. Goals are to: provide data about how common autism is in a specific place and time period; describe the population of children with autism; compare how common autism is in different areas of the country; identify changes in autism occurrence over time; and understand the impact of autism and related conditions in U.S. communities.
	Autism Spectrum Disorder Surveillance of Younger Children (Pilot Alternative Surveillance)	Surveillance	Investigate the feasibility of combining developmental screening and monitoring prevalence of autism for children under the age of 4.
	Centers for Autism and Developmental Disabilities Research and Epidemiology Network	Research	Regional centers of excellence for autism and other developmental disabilities. The primary activity of the network is to conduct the Study to Explore Early Development—a collaborative, multisite epidemiologic study of risk factors for autism.

Table 2. (Continued)

Agency	Activity	Type of activity	Purpose of activity
	Centers for Autism and Developmental Disabilities Research and Epidemiology Data Coordinating Center	Research	Provide a centralized, web-based, automated-workflow system that supports all of the study activities for the Study to Explore Early Development, cited above.
	Georgia Study to Explore Early Development	Research	The Study to Explore Early Development is a multiyear, multisite study in six diverse areas that looks at possible causes of and risks for autism and other developmental delays.
	CDC-Denmark Program	Research	Examine a variety of public health issues, including autism and other developmental disabilities. All studies in this program have a basic activity of either improving existing registries, conducting registry-based studies, or both.
	Minnesota Somali Project (with NIH)c	Surveillance	Investigate reports of elevated prevalence of autism among children born to Somali immigrants living in Minneapolis, Minn.
	Blood Spot Project (award managed by the Department of Defense)	Research	Investigate the relationship between development of autism and cross-reactive antibodies that may cause alterations in fetal brain development. Archived dried blood spots from newborn children who later developed autism and from others who developed normally will be analyzed for specific antibodies. This project is funded by the Department of Defense.
	Learn the Signs. Act Early.[b]	Awareness campaign/ information dissemination	The program is made up of three components: (1) health education campaign promotes awareness of healthy developmental milestones in early childhood, the importance of tracking each child's development, and theimportance of acting early if there are concerns; (2) Act Early Initiative works with state, territorial, and national partners to improve early childhood systems by enhancing collaborative efforts to improve

Agency	Activity	Type of activity	Purpose of activity
			screening and referral to early intervention services and supporting the work of Act Early Ambassadors to promote *Learn the Signs. Act Early.*messages and tools and improve early identification efforts in their state; and (3) research and evaluation improves campaign materials and implementation activities, and increases our understanding of the factors that influence early identification and referral.

Source: GAO analysis of NIH and CDC documents and interviews.

Notes: NIH and CDC funded these autism activities at some point between fiscal years 2006 through 2011, but did not necessarily fund each activity in every fiscal year. In addition to the autism research funded through these activities, NIH funded autism research through other mechanisms, such as through general grant announcements not specific to autism.

[a] In fiscal year 2007 and 2008, respectively, the Collaborative Programs of Excellence in Autism and the Studies to Advance Autism Research and Treatment Network expired. NIH consolidated the funding and goals of these programs into the Autism Centers of Excellence Program.

[b] While these activities are not autism-specific, they include an autism component, such as autism-specific research grants.

[c] This activity was also partially funded by a private organization.

APPENDIX II: LIST OF INTERAGENCY AUTISM COORDINATING COMMITTEE (IACC) REPORTS

Report	Description
Strategic Plan for Autism Spectrum Disorder Research (2009, 2010, 2011)	According to the IACC, the Strategic Plan provides a blueprint for autism research that is advisory to the Department of Health and Human Services and serves as a basis for partnerships with other agencies and private organizations involved in autism research and services. The 2011 Strategic Plan is organized around seven questions asked by individuals with autism and their families (such as "When should I be concerned?"). Each of the seven sections includes a description of what is generally known from autism research for that particular question and what gaps remain, followed by what was learned during the previous year. The report also sets up short- and long-term research objectives based on autism research opportunities. The Combating Autism Act of 2006 (CAA) requires that the Strategic Plan be updated on an annual basis.
Autism Spectrum Disorder Research Portfolio Analysis Report (2008, 2009, 2010)[a]	The Portfolio Analysis features autism project and funding information for certain federal agencies and private organizations. According to officials within the National Institutes of Health Office of Autism Research Coordination (OARC), the agencies and organizations in these reports have been identified by the IACC and OARC as being involved in autism research and have agreed to participate. According to the IACC, the intent of these analysis reports is to better inform the IACC and interested stakeholders about the funding landscape for a particular year. Additionally, the analysis examines the extent to which a particular year's funding and research topics align with the IACC's most recent Strategic Plan. The IACC reports that the Portfolio Analysis may also be used by federal agencies and private research organizations to help guide future funding priorities by outlining current gaps and opportunities in autism research, as well as serving to highlight current activities and research progress. OARC officials told us that they plan to issue the 2011 report in 2013.
Summary of Advances in Autism Spectrum Disorder Research (2007, 2008, 2009, 2010, 2011)	Each year the IACC releases its list of scientific advances in autism research. As reportedby the IACC, the report highlights studies on autism published in the previous year in peer-reviewed journals and selected by members of the IACC.

Report	Description
	The number of studies featured over the years ranges from 20 to 54. The CAA requires that the IACC produce the Summary of Advances annually.
Autism Spectrum Disorder Research Publications Analysis: The Global Landscape of Autism Research[b]	As reported by the IACC, this report describes several key aspects of worldwide autism research publications, which may be used to inform planning and strategic funding decisions for future autism research. Autism-related research articles published between 1980 and 2010 were analyzed to identify historical trends and publication outputs across the seven questions and research areas of the 2011 IACC Strategic Plan. Information found in research publications was also used to assess the institutions conducting autism research, funding organizations supporting the research publications, and the extent of collaboration between authors from different countries and research institutions. Additionally, measures, such as citation counts, were used as an assessment of the impact of the published research. OARC officials told us that there are no plans to update this report annually.

Source: GAO review of IACC and OARC documents.

[a] In 2008 and 2010, OARC, National Institute of Mental Health, prepared this report on behalf of the IACC. In 2009, OARC, National Institute of Mental Health, and Acclaro Research Solutions, Inc., prepared this report on behalf of the IACC.

[b] OARC, National Institute of Mental Health, and Thomson Reuters, Inc., prepared this report on behalf of the IACC.

APPENDIX III: DEPARTMENT OF HEALTH AND HUMAN SERVICES (HHS) FUNDING FOR AUTISM ACTIVITIES FOR FISCAL YEARS 2006 THROUGH 2011

Dollars in millions						
	Fiscal year					
HHS component	**2006**	**2007**	**2008**	**2009**	**2010**	**2011**
Health Resources and Services Administration (HRSA)	$20.0[a]	$19.9[a]	$36.4	$42.0	$47.9	$47.7
National Institutes of Health (NIH)	108.3	126.8	118.1	196.4[b]	217.1[b]	168.7
Centers for Disease Control and Prevention (CDC)	15.1	14.8	16.2	20.4	22.1	21.4
Interagency Autism Coordinating Committee (IACC)	0.2	0.1	1.2	2.6	2.6	2.6
Total[c]	**$143.6**	**$161.6**	**$171.8**	**$261.4**	**$289.7**	**$240.4**

Source: GAO analysis of HRSA, NIH, CDC, and IACC documents and interviews.

Notes: While the Combating Autism Act (CAA) authorized appropriations for HRSA, NIH, CDC, and IACC autism activities, the CAA did not appropriate funds for this purpose. Instead, to fund these activities, HRSA, NIH, and CDC used funds appropriated to the agencies annually through the budget and appropriations process for the purpose of carrying out a variety of programs. As directed by Congress in the annual HHS appropriations acts for fiscal years 2008 through 2011, the Secretary of Health and Human Services transferred funds to NIH's National Institute of Mental Health (NIMH) for the IACC. The IACC also received funds from the annual NIH appropriation for fiscal years 2006 through 2011.

HRSA's totals include autism grant awards, as well as, for example, funding used for HRSA's personnel expenses, travel, supplies, and overhead related to reviewing these grants. NIH's totals include funding for research that is conducted outside of NIH's autism-specific grant announcements. According to NIH officials, much of the autism research funded by NIH is done under general grant announcements soliciting biomedical research. IACC's totals for fiscal years 2008 through 2011 include funding for the Office of Autism Research Coordination within NIMH.

In fiscal year 2008, certain agencies, including HHS agencies, were subject to an across-the-board rescission. All nondefense discretionary programs were subject to an across-the-board rescission in fiscal year 2011. According to HRSA officials, HRSA spent less on its autism activities in these years as a result of the rescissions. NIH officials told us that the agency reduced funding for research grants as a result of the rescissions, but could not measure the precise effect on autism-related grants. According to CDC officials, CDC spent less on its autism activities in fiscal year 2011 as a result of the rescission in that year. In addition, the IACC received less funding in fiscal years 2008 and 2011 as a result of the rescissions.

[a]HRSA's fiscal year 2006 and 2007 funding represents total funding for its Leadership Education in Neurodevelopmental and Other Related Disabilities and Developmental-Behavioral Pediatrics training programs, through which the agency awarded grants that could have had an autism-specific component; however, an autism-specific component was not a requirement of the grants. Beginning in fiscal year 2008, these training programs were required to have an autism-specific component.

[b]NIH's fiscal year 2009 and 2010 funding totals include additional funds appropriated to NIH under the American Recovery and Reinvestment Act of 2009. NIH spent $64 million of these funds in fiscal year 2009 and $57.5 million in fiscal year 2010 on autism activities.

[c]Individual funding entries may not sum to total due to rounding.

APPENDIX IV: COMBATING AUTISM ACT GRANTEES FROM FISCAL YEARS 2008 THROUGH 2011 BY PROGRAM

In fiscal year 2008, in response to the Combating Autism Act, the Health Resources and Services Administration (HRSA) created the *Combating Autism Act Initiative*. Under this initiative, HRSA has a number of programs that fund grants specific to autism. This appendix includes a description of the purpose of each program. Tables 3 through 11 list the grants that have been awarded under each program for fiscal years 2008 through 2011.[1]

Program: Leadership Education in Neurodevelopmental and Other Related Disabilities (LEND) Training Program

The purpose of this program is to improve the health of children who have, or are at risk for developing, neurodevelopmental and other related disabilities by training professionals to assume leadership roles, and to ensure high levels of interdisciplinary clinical competence in an effort to increase diagnosis of or rule out individuals' developmental disabilities, including autism.

Table 3. Leadership Education in Neurodevelopmental and Other Related Disabilities Training Program Grantees from Fiscal Years 2008 through 2011

Dollars					
		Fiscal year			
Grant number	Grantee name	2008 award	2009 award	2010 award	2011 award
T73MC00003	University of Alabama at Birmingham	$755,326	$755,326	$755,326	$680,758
T73MC00008	Children's Hospital of Los Angeles, School of Physical Therapy	818,784	818,784	818,785	650,973
T73MC00013	University of Miami	629,576	729,576	814,576	787,500[a]
T73MC00014	University of Hawaii at Manoa	495,166	595,166	670,166	595,000
T73MC00015	Indiana University, School of Medicine	681,440	681,440	681,440	632,046
T73MC00016	University of Iowa	491,265	591,265	666,265	586,537

Table 3. (Continued)

Dollars					
		Fiscal year			
Grant number	**Grantee name**	**2008 award**	**2009 award**	**2010 award**	**2011 award**
T73MC00019	The Johns Hopkins University	884,277	35,840	0	0
T73MC17245	Kennedy Krieger Children's Hospital, Inc.	0	948,416	1,059,256	850,000
T73MC00020	Children's Hospital (Boston, MA)	755,326	755,326	755,326	745,000[a]
T73MC00022	Curators of University of Missouri at Columbia	393,012	493,012	568,012	574,811
T73MC00023	Board of Regents of the University of Nebraska	612,663	612,663	612,663	622,943
T73MC00024	Trustees of Dartmouth College	651,964	651,964	651,964	848,868
T73MC00025	University of New Mexico Health Sciences Center	527,560	627,560	702,560	680,000
T73MC00027	Albert Einstein College of Medicine	691,265	691,265	691,265	679,299
T73MC00029	University of Rochester	691,265	691,265	691,265	684,028
T73MC00030	University of North Carolina at Chapel Hill	768,691	768,691	798,691	910,004[a]
T73MC00032	University of Cincinnati	766,373	866,373	941,373	800,167
T73MC00033	University of Oklahoma HSC	442,139	542,139	617,139	595,000
T73MC00034	Oregon Health & Sciences University	685,979	785,979	860,979	742,050
T73MC00036	University of Pittsburgh	393,012	493,012	568,012	659,779[a]
T73MC00037	University of South Dakota	432,313	532,313	607,313	602,466[a]
T73MC00038	University of Tennessee at Knoxville	953,109	953,109	953,459	807,500[a]
T73MC00039	University of Vermont	651,964	587,125	651,964	550,000
T73MC00040	Virginia Commonwealth University	451,964	504,798	626,964	584,773
T73MC00041	University of Washington	940,435	940,435	940,435	891,030[a]
T73MC00043	West Virginia University Research Corporation	639,822	639,822	639,822	567,935
T73MC00044	University of Wisconsin at Madison	569,576	669,576	744,576	738,483[a]
T73MC00049	Ohio State University Research Foundation	393,011	493,011	568,011	821,027

Dollars					
		Fiscal year			
Grant number	Grantee name	2008 award	2009 award	2010 award	2011 award
T73MC00050	Vanderbilt University Medical Center	593,012	593,012	623,012	651,500
T73MC00051	The Children's Hospital of Philadelphia	790,966	784,966	790,966	764,391
T73MC00054	University of Utah	755,241	755,241	785,241	823,048[a]
T73MC00056	University of Massachusetts Medical School	604,256	704,256	779,256	685,732
T73MC03181	Children's Research Institute (Washington, DC)	593,012	593,012	593,012	0
T73MC04320	New York Medical College	620,597	720,597	795,597	693,003
T73MC06623	University of Kansas Medical Center Research Institute	743,630	743,630	743,630	641,760
T73MC11044	University of Colorado at Denver	550,000	550,000	550,000	617,500[a]
T73MC11045	University of Arkansas for Medical Sciences	550,000	549,999	549,114	757,995
T73MC11046	University of Connecticut Health Center	550,000	550,000	550,000	0
T73MC11047	University of Illinois at Chicago, College of Medicine	549,999	549,998	550,000	661,752
T73MC12835	Regents of the University of Minnesota	0	450,000	550,000	627,616
T73MC19939	Georgia State University Research Foundation, Inc.	0	0	150,000	545,898
T73MC19940	Board of Regents, Nevada System of Higher Education, on behalf of University of Nevada at Reno	0	0	150,000	508,533
T73MC20662	University of Arizona	0	0	150,000	568,353
T73MC20663	University of Alaska Anchorage	0	0	150,000	530,039
T73MC22233	Medical University of South Carolina	0	0	0	486,440

Table 3. (Continued)

Dollars					
		Fiscal year			
Grant number	Grantee name	2008 award	2009 award	2010 award	2011 award
T73MC22236	The University of Texas Health Science Center at Houston	0	0	0	509,748

Source: GAO analysis of Health Resources and Services Administration (HRSA) information.

[a]Total funding in fiscal year 2011 includes $65,000 of supplemental funds that the grantee received from HRSA's Universal Newborn Hearing Screening program to support additional audiology trainees.

Program: Developmental-Behavioral Pediatrics (DBP) Training Program

The purpose of this program is to train the next generation of leaders in developmental-behavioral pediatrics; and provide pediatric practitioners, residents, and medical students with essential biopsychosocial knowledge and clinical expertise. This program is focused on developmental disabilities, including autism.

Table 4. Developmental-Behavioral Pediatrics Training Program Grantees from Fiscal Years 2008 through 2011

Dollars					
		Fiscal year			
Grant number	Grantee name	2008 award	2009 award	2010 award	2011 award
T77MC00004	Case Western Reserve University	$192,467	$192,467	$192,467	$192,453
T77MC00009	Montefiore Medical Center	192,467	192,467	192,467	192,467
T77MC00011	Children's Hospital (Boston, MA)	192,467	192,467	192,467	192,467
T77MC00012	The Children's Hospital of Philadelphia	229,048	191,943	191,944	191,943
T77MC00015	Boston Medical Center	192,467	192,467	240,467	237,019
T77MC00024	Yale University	209,605	222,467	192,467	192,467

Dollars					
		Fiscal year			
Grant number	Grantee name	2008 award	2009 award	2010 award	2011 award
T77MC09796	Board of Trustees of the Leland Stanford Junior University	142,467	162,467	192,467	192,467
T77MC09797	Rhode Island Hospital	142,467	142,467	192,467	222,467
T77MC09798	University of Arkansas for Medical Sciences, Cancer Research Center	111,143	140,102	144,948	145,000
T77MC09799	University of Oklahoma, Health Sciences Center	142,467	142,467	172,467	142,467

Source: GAO analysis of Health Resources and Services Administration (HRSA) information.

Program: National Combating Autism Interdisciplinary Training Resource Center

The purpose of this program is to improve the health of children who have, or are at risk for developing, autism and other developmental disabilities by providing technical assistance to LEND and DBP programs to better train professionals to utilize valid and reliable screening tools for diagnosing or ruling out autism, and provide evidence-based interventions for children.

Table 5. National Combating Autism Interdisciplinary Training Resource Center Grantees from Fiscal Years 2008 through 2011

Dollars					
		Fiscal year			
Grant number	Grantee name	2008 award	2009 award	2010 award	2011 award
UA5MC11068	Association of University Centers on Disabilities	$487,641	$547,641	$637,314	$784,641

Source: GAO analysis of Health Resources and Services Administration (HRSA) information.

Note: Funding in fiscal years 2010 and 2011 includes supplemental funds of $89,673 and $147,000, respectively, which the grantee received from HRSA's Universal Newborn Hearing Screening program to support audiology training within HRSA's Leadership Education in Neurodevelopmental and Other Related Disabilities training program.

Program: Autism Intervention Research Program and Autism Intervention Secondary Data Analysis Studies Program

The purpose of this program is to support research on evidence-based practices for interventions to improve the health and well-being of children and adolescents with autism and other developmental disabilities. The Autism Intervention Secondary Data Analysis Studies Program utilizes the analysis of existing secondary data.

Table 6. Autism Intervention Research Program and Autism Intervention Secondary Data Analysis Studies Program Grantees from Fiscal Years 2008 through 2011

Dollars					
		Fiscal year			
Grant number	**Grantee name**	**2008 award**	**2009 award**	**2010 award**	**2011 award**
R40MC15593	University of Colorado at Denver	$0	$393,024	$400,000	$0
R40MC15594	Kennedy Krieger Institute, Inc.	0	393,024	400,000	0
R40MC15595	University of North Carolina at Chapel Hill	0	93,533	0	0
R40MC15596	Boston Medical Center	0	393,019	399,994	0
R40MC15597	University of New Hampshire	0	393,024	400,000	0
R40MC15598	Brandeis University	0	334,359	291,635	0
R40MC16396	University of Massachusetts at Boston	0	100,000	0	0
R40MC17158	University of North Carolina at Chapel Hill	0	0	100,000	0
R40MC17170	Georgia State University Research Foundation, Inc.	0	0	100,000	0
R40MC19925	The General Hospital Corporation	0	0	256,917	294,647
R40MC19926	The Curators of the University of Missouri	0	0	184,288	188,378
R40MC19927	Brandeis University	0	0	98,962	0
R40MC19928	Boston Medical Center Corporation	0	0	299,906	298,072
R40MC20171	Georgetown University	0	0	299,993	299,955
R40MC20172	University of Connecticut Health Center	0	0	300,000	300,000
R40MC20444	West Virginia University Research Corporation	0	0	296,372	296,146
R40MC20611	Health Research, Inc. / New York State Department of Health	0	0	300,000	300,000

Dollars					
		Fiscal year			
Grant number	Grantee name	2008 award	2009 award	2010 award	2011 award
R40MC22641	Regents of the University of California	0	0	0	285,177
R40MC22642	Regents of the University of California	0	0	0	99,988
R40MC22643	University of Colorado at Denver	0	0	0	300,000
R40MC22644	University of Iowa	0	0	0	299,972
R40MC22645	University of Massachusetts	0	0	0	300,000
R40MC22646	University of Massachusetts at Boston	0	0	0	100,000
R40MC22647	University of North Carolina at Chapel Hill	0	0	0	100,000
R40MC22648	University of North Carolina at Chapel Hill	0	0	0	299,997

Source: GAO analysis of Health Resources and Services Administration (HRSA) information.

Program: Autism Intervention Research Network on Physical Health

The purpose of this program is to establish and maintain a network infrastructure designed to be the platform from which to conduct research on evidence-based practices for interventions to improve the physical health and well-being of individuals with autism and other developmental disabilities; develop evidence-based guidelines and validate tools for interventions; and disseminate critical information on its research findings, guidelines, and tools.

Table 7. Autism Intervention Research Network on Physical Health Grantees from Fiscal Years 2008 through 2011

Dollars					
		Fiscal year			
Grant number	Grantee name	2008 award	2009 award	2010 award	2011 award
UA3MC 11054	The General Hospital Corporation	$3,999,342	$3,997,824	$3,651,425	$3,999,847

Source: GAO analysis of Health Resources and Services Administration (HRSA) information.

Program: Autism Intervention Research Network on Behavioral Health

The purpose of this program is to establish and maintain a network infrastructure designed to be the platform from which to conduct research on evidence-based interventions to improve the behavioral, mental, social, or cognitive health, or a mix of those, and well-being of children and adolescents with autism and other developmental disabilities; develop evidence-based guidelines and validate tools for interventions; and disseminate critical information on its research findings, guidelines, and tools.

Table 8. Autism Intervention Research Network on Behavioral Health Grantees from Fiscal Years 2008 through 2011

Dollars					
		Fiscal year			
Grant number	**Grantee name**	**2008 award**	**2009 award**	**2010 award**	**2011 award**
UA3MC 11055	Regents of the University of California	$2,000,000	$1,930,288	$1,989,276	$2,000,000

Source: GAO analysis of Health Resources and Services Administration (HRSA) information.

Program: Developmental-Behavioral Pediatrics Research Network

The purpose of this program is to establish a multicenter scientific and clinical research network that will promote coordinated research activities and address health issues. The program is intended to build a developmental behavioral pediatric research infrastructure that supports multidisciplinary research, focuses on the translation of research to practice, and provides the environment in which to train a new generation of developmental behavioral pediatric researchers.

Table 9. Developmental-Behavioral Pediatrics Research Network Grantees from Fiscal Years 2008 through 2011

Dollars					
		Fiscal year			
Grant number	Grantee name	2008 award	2009 award	2010 award	2011 award
UA3MC20218	The Children's Hospital of Philadelphia	$0	$0	$200,000	$220,000

Source: GAO analysis of Health Resources and Services Administration (HRSA) information.

Program: State Implementation and Planning Grants

The purpose of this program is to improve access to comprehensive, coordinated health care and related services by implementing state plans to improve the system of services.[2]

Table 10. State Implementation and Planning Grants Grantees from Fiscal Years 2008 through 2011

Dollars					
		Fiscal year			
Grant number	Grantee name	2008 award	2009 award	2010 award	2011 award
H6MMC11059[a]	The Curators of the University of Missouri	$297,957	$295,703	$467,729	$0
H6MMC11061[a]	Utah Department of Health	300,000	300,000	497,757	0
H6MMC11062	The Hope School (Springfield, IL)	300,000	300,000	300,000	0
H6MMC11063	Wisconsin Department of Health & Family Services	300,000	300,000	300,000	0
H6MMC11064[a]	State of Alaska, Department of Health & Social Services	300,000	300,000	497,757	0
H6MMC11065[a]	State of Washington Department of Health	300,000	300,000	497,757	0
H6MMC15102	Rhode Island Department of Health	0	300,000	300,000	0
H6MMC15103	University of New Mexico Health Sciences Center	0	300,000	300,000	0

Table 10. (Continued)

Dollars					
		Fiscal year			
Grant number	**Grantee name**	**2008 award**	**2009 award**	**2010 award**	**2011 award**
H6MMC15104	Health Research, Inc. / New York State Department of Health	0	300,000	300,000	0
H6MMC20326	Vermont State Department of Health	0	0	272,463	300,000
H6MMC20327	Hawaii Pediatric Association Research & Education Foundation	0	0	272,463	300,000
H6MMC20328	Statewide Parent Advocacy Network of New Jersey	0	0	272,463	300,000
H6MMC20329	Maine Department of Health and Human Services	0	0	272,463	300,000
H6MMC22710	Georgia State University Research Foundation	0	0	0	75,000
H6MMC22711	Tennessee Disability Coalition	0	0	0	75,000
H6MMC22712	The Parents' Place of Maryland	0	0	0	75,000
H6MMC22713	University of Delaware	0	0	0	74,999
H6MMC22737	Autism Society of Colorado	0	0	0	243,092
H6MMC22738	Connecticut Department of Public Health	0	0	0	243,092
H6MMC22739	Minot State University	0	0	0	243,092
H6MMC22740	University of Southern Mississippi	0	0	0	243,092
H6MMC22849	Ohio Department of Developmental Disabilities	0	0	0	243,092

Source: GAO analysis of Health Resources and Services Administration (HRSA) information.

[a]Totals for this grantee in fiscal year 2010 include supplemental funding to expand its implementation of the Centers for Disease Control and Prevention's (CDC) *Learn the Signs. Act Early.* campaign. This supplement is funded through an interagency agreement between HRSA and CDC.

Program: State Public Health Coordinating Center

The program purpose is to improve the health of children who have, or are at risk for developing, autism and other developmental disabilities by coordinating with the state demonstration grantees; and by developing a strategy for defining, supporting, and monitoring the role of state public health agencies in assuring early and timely identification, diagnosis, and intervention.

Table 11. State Public Health Coordinating Center Grantees from Fiscal Years 2008 through 2011

Dollars					
		Fiscal year			
Grant number	**Grantee name**	**2008 award**	**2009 award**	**2010 award**	**2011 award**
U01MC 11069	Association of Maternal & Child Health Programs	$250,000	$250,000	$275,000	$275,000

Source: GAO analysis of Health Resources and Services Administration (HRSA) information.

End Notes

[1] CDC's most recent estimates are based on data collected in 14 areas of the United States. CDC's estimate of autism prevalence in 2012 is based on data from calendar year 2008, and the 2009 estimate is based on data from calendar year 2006.

[2] In this report, we use the term "autism" to refer to autism spectrum disorders.

[3] Pub. L. No. 109-416, 120 Stat. 2821 (Dec. 19, 2006).

[4] These activities were reauthorized and additional funding was authorized through fiscal year 2014 under the Combating Autism Reauthorization Act of 2011. Pub. L. No. 111-32, 125 Stat. 361 (Sept. 30, 2011).

[5] A subsequent report will examine the involvement of federal agencies in autism activities and the coordination of these activities.

[6] HRSA was included in the review because the CAA requires the Secretary of Health and Human Services to establish various autism activities, and HRSA carries out these activities.

[7] This guidance includes: HHS, *Awarding Agency Grants Administration Manual* (2007); HHS, *Grants Policy Statement* (2007); and HRSA, Office of Federal Assistance Management, Division of Grants Management Operations, *Operational & Procedures Manual* (2009).

[8] Our sample is too small to generalize the results to the 110 CAA grantees as a whole; however, our sample is representative of the population of CAA grantees.

[9] Agency staff use the EHB to award grants, review information related to CAA grants, and monitor CAA grantees' performance. Grantees upload information pertaining to their grant—such as required reports—and agency staff can indicate their review and approval of this information, in the EHB. While the submission of performance reports—a report grantees submit annually with performance and budget information—is documented in the

EHB, it is not possible to view these reports in the EHB. These reports can be viewed in the Discretionary Grant Information System—a system that regularly collects program and performance measure data, including performance reports, submitted by grantees. We reviewed files relating to grants awarded in fiscal years 2008 through 2011 that were included in these two data systems as of early October 2012.

[10] A developmental disability is a chronic condition caused by mental impairment, physical impairment, or both that begins any time during prenatal development up to age 22 and usually persists throughout a person's life. Individuals with developmental disabilities have substantial functional limitations in at least three major life activities such as language, mobility, learning, self-help, and independent living. Developmental disabilities may include cerebral palsy, hearing loss, intellectual disability, and vision impairment.

[11] A cooperative agreement is an alternative assistance instrument used instead of a grant whenever substantial federal involvement with the recipient during performance is anticipated.

[12] Pub. L. No. 106-310, 114 Stat. 1101 (Oct. 17, 2000). We previously reported on federal autism activities under the Children's Health Act. See GAO, *Federal Autism Activities: Funding for Research Has Increased, but Agencies Need to Resolve Surveillance Challenges*, GAO-06-700 (Washington, D.C.: July 19, 2006).

[13] The CAA directs the Secretary of Health and Human Services to undertake autism education, early detection, and intervention activities, subject to the availability of federal funding; and HRSA and CDC carry out these activities. The CAA directives are: provide information and education on autism and other developmental disabilities to increase public awareness of developmental milestones; promote research into the development and validation of reliable screening tools for autism and other developmental disabilities, and disseminate information regarding those screening tools; promote early screening of individuals at higher risk for autism and other developmental disabilities as early as practicable, given evidence-based screening techniques and interventions; increase the number of individuals who are able to confirm or rule out a diagnosis of autism and other developmental disabilities; increase the number of individuals able to provide evidence-based interventions for individuals diagnosed with autism or other developmental disabilities; and, promote the use of evidence-based interventions for individuals at higher risk for autism and other developmental disabilities as early as practicable.

[14] HRSA spent approximately $19.9 million on the LEND and DBP training programs in fiscal year 2007. In fiscal year 2008, when the *Combating Autism Act Initiative* was implemented, HRSA spent approximately $25.8 million on the LEND and DBP training programs.

[15] The states that received state implementation and planning grants are Alaska, Colorado, Connecticut, Delaware, Georgia, Hawaii, Illinois, Maine, Maryland, Mississippi, Missouri, New Jersey, New Mexico, New York, North Dakota, Ohio, Rhode Island, Tennessee, Utah, Vermont, Washington, and Wisconsin.

[16] In contrast to the requirement contained in the Children's Health Act, however, the CAA directs NIH and CDC to undertake these activities subject to the availability of appropriations.

[17] *See*, for example, Public Health Service Act, § 301 (codified at 42 U.S.C. § 241) (providing NIH broad authority to award grants to public and private institutions to conduct scientific research).

[18] The CAA specified that the IACC include certain federal members, such as officials from CDC, NIH, and the Department of Education. It also required the Secretary to appoint a minimum number of nonfederal members, which must include at least one person with

autism; at least one parent or legal guardian of a person with autism; and at least one representative of a leading research, advocacy, or service organization for individuals with autism. The Children's Health Act did not require that nonfederal entities or officials from the Department of Education be included as IACC members. However, the Children's Health Act authorized the Secretary of Health and Human Services to appoint parents or legal guardians of individuals with autism to the committee. Prior to the enactment of the CAA, the committee included four nonfederal members.

[19] The CAA also requires the IACC to make recommendations to the Secretary of Health and Human Services on any changes to federal activities, including recommendations made in the strategic plan on autism research.

[20] Prior to the CAA, the IACC produced a research matrix that NIH officials viewed as a comprehensive list of autism research goals. It also issued an autism roadmap that provided a synthesis of issues and challenges related to services for individuals with autism and a set of performance measures and recommendations for improving services.

[21] In addition, on behalf of the Secretary of Health and Human Services, OARC produced a report to Congress on autism activities as required by the CAA. See HHS, OARC, NIH, *Report to Congress on Activities Related to Autism Spectrum Disorder and Other Developmental Disabilities Under the Combating Autism Act of 2006 (FY 2006 – FY 2009)* (Rockville, Md.: December 2010, revised April 2011).

[22] While the CAA authorized appropriations for HRSA, NIH, and CDC autism activities, the CAA did not appropriate funds for this purpose. Instead, to fund these activities, HRSA, NIH, and CDC used funds appropriated to the agencies annually through the budget and appropriations process for the purpose of carrying out a variety of programs.

[23] In fiscal year 2008, certain agencies, including HHS agencies, were subject to an across-the-board rescission. All nondefense discretionary programs were subject to an across-the-board rescission in fiscal year 2011. According to HRSA officials, HRSA spent less on its autism activities in these years as a result of the rescissions. NIH officials told us that the agency reduced funding for research grants as a result of the rescissions, but could not measure the precise effect on autism-related grants. According to CDC officials, CDC spent less on its autism activities in fiscal year 2011 as a result of the rescission in that year. In addition, the IACC received less funding in fiscal years 2008 and 2011 as a result of the rescissions.

[24] HRSA issued these grants as part of its *Combating Autism Act Initiative*. For the purpose of this report we are referring to the programs and grantees in HRSA's *Combating Autism Act Initiative* as CAA grantees or CAA programs.

[25] The annual federal financial reports were formerly called financial status reports. A budget period is the interval of time (usually 12 months each) into which a project period is divided for budgetary and funding purposes. The project period refers to the total period for which support of a project has been programmatically approved.

[26] Grantees who submit a competing continuation application include a progress report summarizing progress made over the entire previous project period along with their application. Grantees who do not reapply for a grant, and complete the period of project support from HRSA, must submit a comprehensive final report. This report covers the last year of the project period and includes information on progress over all years of the project period.

[27] HRSA started requiring mid-project reports of grantees in its Autism Intervention Research and Autism Intervention Secondary Data Analysis Studies Programs in fiscal year 2010. Because Autism Intervention Secondary Data Analysis Studies Program grants are 1-year grants, the reports are referred to as mid-year progress reports.

[28] The research networks are the Autism Intervention Research Network on Physical Health, Autism Intervention Research Network on Behavioral Health, and Developmental-Behavioral Pediatric Research Network.

[29] Progress reports that are submitted as part of competing continuation applications are reviewed with the application. HRSA staff use a checklist when reviewing the application.

[30] HRSA grantees request funds that they have available at any time during the budget period through the use of an online form that is submitted to the HRSA Payment Management System. The Payment Management System keeps track of how often and what amount of funds are withdrawn by the grantee during the course of the budget period.

[31] Our unbiased random sample of 22 grantees consisted of 11 training grantees, 7 research grantees, and 4 state implementation and planning grantees. This sample is representative of the 110 CAA grantees. The grantees in our sample received about $28 million—about 17 percent—of the total awards CAA grantees received from fiscal years 2008 through 2011. HRSA officials stated that no CAA grantees were high-risk grantees, and we found this to be accurate for the grantees we reviewed. "High risk" is used to describe a grantee that is at risk of financial failure or failure to perform based on a history of poor performance or poor business practices, financial instability, or inadequate management systems.

[32] This includes 46 federal financial reports, 54 progress reports, 4 mid-project progress reports, and 2 comprehensive final reports. This count includes one annual federal financial report per grantee per year. Grantees are allowed to revise and resubmit their federal financial report if they find that information needs to be corrected.

[33] The question in the checklist is: "Are there any areas of concern: programmatic, budgetary, or other?"

[34] In one instance, the grantee had not yet submitted the revised report at the time of our review.

[35] The notice of award is the official document that states the terms, conditions, and amount of a grant award and is signed by the official who is authorized to obligate funds on behalf of HRSA. A notice of award shows the amount of federal funds available to the grantee and is issued at the start of each budget period. A revised notice of award may be issued during a budget period to effect an action resulting in a change in the amount of support or other change in the terms and conditions of award, such as a carryover of funds.

[36] According to HRSA officials, HRSA staff began using a checklist to indicate their review and approval of prior-approval requests at the end of calendar year 2009. Prior to this, the issuance of a new notice of award indicated HRSA review and approval of such requests. We reviewed one carryover request related to an award in fiscal year 2010 that did not have a review checklist in the EHB; however, a new notice of award indicated that the carryover request had been approved.

[37] Grantees in HRSA's Autism Intervention Research and Autism Intervention Secondary Data Analysis Studies Programs are required to have a web-based site visit at project end.

[38] Performance reports include financial forms, project abstracts and other grant summary data, and performance measures. Grantees submit initial performance reports at the beginning of the project period, annual performance reports after the end of each budget year, and project period end performance reports after the end of the project period.

[39] HRSA expects to submit this report to Congress in the middle of calendar year 2013.

[40] HRSA, Maternal and Child Health Bureau, *Operations Manual, Combating Autism Act Initiative* (Rockville, Md.: December 2012).

[41] HHS guidance indicates that a program-wide approach to monitoring grantees must be established and reviewed at least annually to determine if the approach needs to be

modified. This annual review should be documented, as appropriate, in the program information file. HHS, *Awarding Agency Grants Administration Manual.*

End Notes for Appendix IV

[1] The fiscal years in tables 3 through 11 are based on the start date of the budget period for which the grant was awarded. The budget period for some of these grantees is from July 1 through June 31, and the budget period for other grantees is from September 1 through August 31. Under its *Combating Autism Act Initiative,* HRSA also provided supplemental funding to two existing cooperative agreements. A cooperative agreement is an alternative assistance instrument used instead of a grant whenever substantial federal involvement with the recipient during performance is anticipated. The first supplement is to provide technical assistance to grantees under one of HRSA's *Combating Autism Act Initiative* Programs—Leadership Education in Neurodevelopmental and Other Related Disabilities. The grantee is Georgetown University in Washington, D.C., and the grantee received $22,000 and $43,550 in fiscal years 2010 and 2011, respectively. The second supplement is to examine current knowledge, research gaps, and methodological challenges about the life-course trajectory of individuals with autism, and develop a lifecourse-focused autism research agenda. The grantee is the Regents of the University of California at Los Angeles and the grantee received $30,785 in fiscal year 2011.

[2] This program comprises: State Implementation Grants for Improving Services for Children and Youth with Autism Spectrum Disorder and other Developmental Disabilities, and State Planning Grants for Improving Services for Children and Youth with Autism Spectrum Disorder and other Developmental Disabilities.

In: The Combating Autism Act
Editor: Deryck Harlow
ISBN: 978-1-63321-128-5

Chapter 3

FEDERAL AUTISM ACTIVITIES: BETTER DATA AND MORE COORDINATION NEEDED TO HELP AVOID THE POTENTIAL FOR UNNECESSARY DUPLICATION*

United States Government Accountability Office

WHY GAO DID THIS STUDY

Autism—a developmental disorder involving communication and social impairment—is an important public health concern. From fiscal years 2008 through 2012, 12 federal agencies awarded at least $1.4 billion to support autism research and other autism-related activities. The CAA directed the IACC to coordinate HHS autism activities and monitor all federal autism activities. It also required the IACC to develop and annually update a strategic plan for autism research. This plan is organized into 7 research areas that contain specific objectives.

GAO was asked to examine federal autism efforts. In this report, GAO (1) analyzes the extent to which federal agencies fund potentially duplicative autism research, and (2) assesses the extent to which IACC and agencies coordinate and monitor federal autism activities. GAO analyzed agencies' data

* This is an edited, reformatted and augmented version of United States Government Accountability Office Publication, No. GAO-14-16, dated November 2013.

and documents, and interviewed federal agency officials and select nonfederal IACC members.

WHAT GAO RECOMMENDS

GAO is recommending that (1) HHS improve the usefulness of IACC data to enhance coordination and monitoring of federal autism activities, and DOD, Education, HHS, and NSF improve their coordination of autism research. HHS disagreed with the first recommendation stating that it was already making adequate efforts. The agencies supported the need for improved coordination but, except for DOD, disputed that any duplication occurs. GAO continues to believe the recommendations are warranted as discussed in the report.

WHAT GAO FOUND

Eighty-four percent of the autism research projects funded by federal agencies had the potential to be duplicative. Of the 1,206 autism research projects funded by federal agencies from fiscal years 2008 through 2012, 1,018 projects were potentially duplicative because the projects were categorized to the same objectives in the Interagency Autism Coordinating Committee's (IACC) strategic plan. Funding similar research on the same topic is sometimes appropriate—for example, for purposes of replicating or corroborating results—but in some instances, funding similar research may lead to unnecessary duplication. The potentially duplicative research projects included those funded by the Department of Defense (DOD), Department of Education (Education), National Science Foundation (NSF), and agencies within the Department of Health and Human Services (HHS)—Administration for Children and Families, Agency for Healthcare Research and Quality, Centers for Disease Control and Prevention (CDC), Centers for Medicare & Medicaid Services, Health Resources and Services Administration, National Institutes of Health (NIH), and the Substance Abuse and Mental Health Services Administration. Each agency funded at least 1 autism research project in the same strategic plan objective as another agency. For example, 5 agencies awarded approximately $15.2 million for 20 autism research projects related to 1 objective to test methods to improve dissemination, implementation, and sustainability of evidence-based interventions, services, and supports in diverse community settings.

The IACC's and federal agencies' efforts to coordinate and monitor federal autism activities were limited. The IACC—composed of federal and nonfederal members—met regularly and issued several reports, such as a strategic plan and portfolio analysis—a report that provides information on autism research projects, organized by the strategic plan objectives. The IACC has also released a companion database to its portfolio analysis. However, IACC members provided mixed views on the usefulness of the IACC's meetings, strategic plan, and portfolio analysis in aiding coordination and monitoring. While three agencies— CDC, DOD, and NIH—regularly used the committee's strategic plan and portfolio analysis, others did not. Shortcomings in the data the IACC used for its portfolio analysis limited its ability to coordinate HHS autism activities and monitor federal autism activities—as required by the Combating Autism Act of 2006 (CAA). For example, GAO found that the data used by the IACC was outdated, not tracked over time, inconsistent, and incomplete. These weaknesses limited the IACC's ability to monitor its progress on its coordination and monitoring efforts—which, in prior work, GAO established as a best practice for inter-agency collaboration, as well as a federal internal control standard. In addition, these weaknesses limited agencies' ability to use these data to identify coordination opportunities and avoid the potential for unnecessary duplication. Such information is important because of the involvement of multiple agencies. Lastly, apart from their participation on the IACC, there were limited instances of agencies coordinating, and agencies did not have robust or routine procedures for monitoring federal autism activities. Per federal internal control standards, agencies should establish a means of communicating with other agencies; this is important to maximize the efficiency of the federal autism investment and minimize the potential for unnecessary duplication.

ABBREVIATIONS

ACF	Administration for Children and Families
ACL	Administration for Community Living
AHRQ	Agency for Healthcare Research and Quality
CAA	Combating Autism Act of 2006
CDC	Centers for Disease Control and Prevention
CMS	Centers for Medicare & Medicaid Services

DOD	Department of Defense
EPA	Environmental Protection Agency
HHS	Department of Health and Human Services
HRSA	Health Resources and Services Administration
IACC	Interagency Autism Coordinating Committee
LEND	Leadership Education in Neurodevelopmental and Other Related Disabilities
NIH	National Institutes of Health
NSF	National Science Foundation
OARC	Office of Autism Research Coordination
RePORTER	Research Portfolio Online Reporting Tools Expenditures and Results
SAMHSA	Substance Abuse and Mental Health Services Administration

November 20, 2013

Congressional Requesters

Autism is an important public health concern, according to the Centers for Disease Control and Prevention (CDC)—an agency within the Department of Health and Human Services (HHS). CDC estimates suggest that the prevalence of autism is increasing, and that at least 1 in 88 children in the United States have been identified as having autism.[1] Autism is a complex developmental disorder that begins during early childhood, characterized by impaired social interactions, problems with verbal and nonverbal communication, and repetitive behaviors, or by severely limited activities and interests. What is commonly known as autism is a group of disorders known as autism spectrum disorder that can range from mild to more severe in their symptoms.[2]

From fiscal year 2008 through fiscal year 2012, 12 federal agencies funded autism research and other autism-related activities.[3,4] For example, agencies funded research to identify the causes of autism, as well as training for health care professionals on identifying and diagnosing autism. From fiscal year 2008 through fiscal year 2012, these agencies spent at least $1.4 billion on autism research and other autism-related activities.

To address growing concern about the increasing prevalence of autism and to stimulate research into possible autism causes and interventions, the

Combating Autism Act of 2006 (CAA) was enacted in December of that year.[5] The CAA reauthorized the Interagency Autism Coordinating Committee (IACC), which is a federal advisory committee that was initially established under the Children's Health Act of 2000.[6] The CAA directs the IACC to coordinate all autism activities within HHS and to monitor federal activities related to autism. The IACC includes members representing 10 federal agencies—8 agencies within HHS, the Department of Defense (DOD), and the Department of Education (Education). In addition, there are 14 nonfederal members who represent individuals with autism and parents of children with autism; as well as members of the autism advocacy, research, and service-provider communities.[7] The CAA also requires the IACC to develop and annually update a strategic plan for autism research.[8] The strategic plan is organized into 7 research areas that contain specific short- and long-term research objectives. The National Institutes of Health (NIH)—an agency within HHS—created the Office of Autism Research Coordination (OARC) to provide administrative support to the IACC. On behalf of the IACC, OARC periodically collects data from agencies on the autism research they fund and helps agencies categorize this research to the specific strategic plan objectives.

Having multiple agencies involved in autism research and other autism-related activities can be advantageous, as agencies may be able to tailor programs to suit their specific missions and needs. In some instances, funding similar research on the same topic is appropriate and necessary; for example, for purposes of replicating or corroborating prior research results. However, it is important that agencies monitor federal autism efforts and coordinate similar actions to maximize their effectiveness and efficiency and avoid the potential for unnecessary duplication. You asked us to provide information on the extent to which federal autism activities are duplicative and the extent to which federal autism activities are coordinated. In this report, we

1) analyze the extent to which federal agencies fund potentially duplicative autism research and other autism-related activities, and
2) assess the extent to which the IACC and agencies coordinate and monitor federal autism activities.

To analyze the extent to which federal agencies fund potentially duplicative autism research and other autism-related activities, we first identified the agencies funding such research and activities and collected data on the nature of the research or activities and the associated funding amounts. Specifically, we identified those federal agencies that funded autism research projects and autism-related activities from fiscal years 2008 to 2011 through interviews, review of related documentation, and database searches. We considered a federal agency to have funded autism research or an autism-related activity if the research project or activity was autism-specific or had an autism-specific component, and was supported by federal funds awarded under mechanisms such as grants, cooperative agreements, or contracts; or was research conducted by scientists in government laboratories, known as intramural research.[9] We compared the agency data we collected to information collected by OARC on behalf of the IACC. We also included any agencies and the related research projects they funded in fiscal year 2012, as identified in data that agencies submitted to OARC.[10]

Next, to determine potential duplication in autism research, we identified research projects that were categorized to the same strategic plan objectives. For those projects that were not categorized to a specific objective, but were categorized to one of the seven research areas, we assessed duplication based on whether they were categorized to the same research area. Determining that projects were categorized to the same strategic plan objective or research area suggests potential, but not actual duplication. Determining actual duplication for research projects would require a more extensive review of voluminous and scientific data, and was beyond the scope of this study.

Finally, we assessed whether there was actual duplication of non-research autism-related activities using the framework we established in our previous work. This framework considers duplication to have occurred when two or more agencies fund the same activities that target the same users.[11] To determine if the activities and targeted users were the same, we reviewed each activity's purpose and strategy for achieving that purpose and reviewed the targeted population of the activities. We assessed the reliability of the data we obtained by comparing agency data to data collected by OARC, following up with agency officials regarding discrepancies in the data, and gathering information from agencies on the internal controls they use when maintaining their data. We found the data reliable for our purposes. For more information on our scope and methodology for determining whether federal agencies fund potentially duplicative autism research and other autism-related activities, see appendix I.

To assess the extent to which the IACC and agencies coordinate and monitor federal autism activities, we reviewed IACC documents, including the strategic plan. We also interviewed OARC officials and officials from 10 federal agencies. Eight of these agencies were IACC members. The other 2 agencies were not IACC members, but funded autism-related research between fiscal years 2008 and 2012. We also interviewed select nonfederal IACC members.[12] Our review of documents and interviews allowed us to determine the methods used by the IACC to coordinate HHS activities and monitor federal autism activities. It also allowed us to determine how agencies coordinate and monitor federal autism activities apart from the IACC to prevent unnecessary duplication. We assessed the IACC's and agencies' coordination and monitoring activities against criteria established by our prior work, including key practices for interagency coordination and collaboration, and federal internal control standards related to communicating with external entities, including other agencies, and measuring progress on organizational efforts, such as those established through strategic plans.[13]

We conducted this performance audit from December 2012 to November 2013 in accordance with generally accepted government auditing standards. Those standards require that we plan and perform the audit to obtain sufficient, appropriate evidence to provide a reasonable basis for our findings based on our audit objectives. We believe that the evidence obtained provides a reasonable basis for our findings and conclusions based on our audit objectives.

BACKGROUND

Autism—a complex and pervasive developmental disability—begins during early childhood, although signs and symptoms vary.[14] According to CDC, autism begins before age 3 and lasts throughout a person's life. Some children show signs of autism within the first few months of life. In others, symptoms might not be apparent until 24 months or later. Still other children with autism seem to develop typically until 18 to 24 months of age and then stop gaining new skills or lose the skills they had. Signs and symptoms of autism include a child not responding to his or her name by 12 months; not pointing at objects to show interest by 14 months; avoiding eye contact and wanting to be alone; repeating words or phrases over and over; and flapping hands, rocking, or spinning in circles. Individuals with autism might have problems with showing or talking about their feelings and might also have trouble understanding the feelings of others.

Diagnosing autism can be difficult, as there is no medical diagnostic test available. As a result, doctors consider a child's behavior and development to make a clinical diagnosis. By age 2, a diagnosis by an experienced professional can be considered very reliable. However, according to CDC, most children do not receive a diagnosis until after age 4. There is no single known cause of autism, but a variety of factors are suspected of causing or contributing to autism, including environmental, biological, and genetic factors. While there is no known cure, research shows that early intervention treatment services can greatly improve a child's development. Because of the complexity of this disorder, individuals with autism have diverse needs for medical and mental health care, as well as an array of educational and social services.

To address growing concern about the increasing prevalence of autism and to stimulate research into possible autism causes and interventions, the CAA was enacted in December 2006. The CAA amended sections of the Children's Health Act of 2000—which required HHS to conduct activities related to autism research, surveillance, and coordination—and authorized the expansion of HHS's autism activities and funding for such activities through fiscal year 2011. The Combating Autism Reauthorization Act of 2011 reauthorized these activities and authorized funding through fiscal year 2014.

In 2008, NIH created OARC to provide administrative support to the IACC. OARC assists the IACC in fulfilling the IACC's responsibilities established by the CAA. Among other things, it conducts analyses and prepares reports for the IACC; assists with the IACC's strategic planning and monitoring of autism activities; coordinates cross-agency efforts; gathers public input to inform the work of the IACC; disseminates information about the work of the IACC and autism research activities to the public, Congress, and other government agencies; and provides logistical support for IACC meetings. In addition to assisting the IACC, OARC produced a report to Congress on federal autism activities on behalf of the Secretary of Health and Human Services, as required by the CAA.[15]

The 12 federal agencies that funded autism research and other autism-related activities between fiscal years 2008 and 2012 were DOD; Education; the Environmental Protection Agency (EPA); the National Science Foundation (NSF); and 8 agencies within HHS—Administration for Children and Families (ACF), Administration for Community Living (ACL), Agency for Healthcare Research and Quality (AHRQ), CDC, Centers for Medicare & Medicaid Services (CMS), Health Resources and Services Administration (HRSA), NIH, and Substance Abuse and Mental Health Services Administration (SAMHSA). With the exception of EPA, NSF, and SAMHSA, these agencies have representatives on the IACC.[16] Eleven of these 12 agencies awarded approximately $1.2 billion to fund autism research projects from fiscal years 2008 through 2012, as shown in figure 1.[17] NIH was the biggest supporter of autism research, awarding approximately 81 percent of the funding from fiscal years 2008 through 2012.

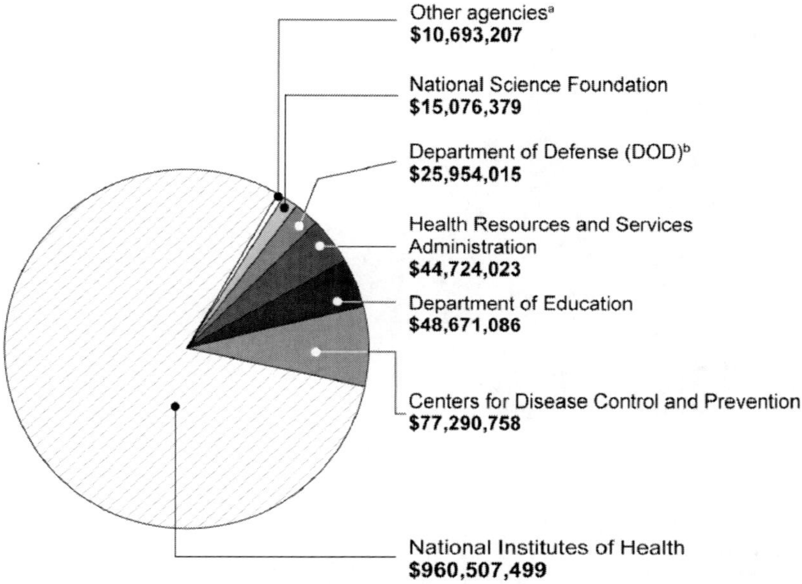

Source: GAO analysis of data from federal agencies that funded autism research.

[a]Other agencies are Administration for Children and Families (1 project), Agency for Healthcare Research and Quality (5 projects), Centers for Medicare & Medicaid Services (4 projects), Environmental Protection Agency (1 project), and Substance Abuse and Mental Health Services (1 project).

[b]DOD's fiscal year 2012 appropriation for its medical research programs, including autism, was available for obligation through the end of fiscal year 2013—September 30, 2013. At the time of our review, DOD had not submitted data on its fiscal year 2012 research projects in response to the Office of Autism Research Coordination's request. As a result, the funding amount for DOD does not include DOD's funding for fiscal year 2012 autism research.

Figure 1. Federal Funds Awarded for Autism Research Projects, Fiscal Years 2008 through 2012.

In addition, of the 12 agencies, 5 awarded approximately $204 million for non-research autism-related activities from fiscal years 2008 through 2011, as shown in figure 2.

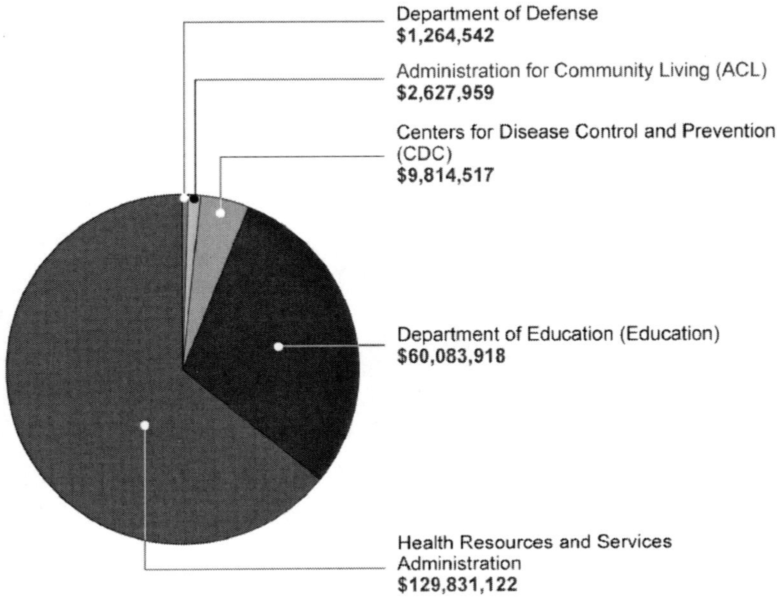

Source: GAO analysis of data from federal agencies that funded autism-related non-research activities.

Notes: Most of Education's activities included projects that were not related to autism. The funding presented for Education represents the funding amounts that supported projects that were autism-specific or had a component to them that was autism-specific.

With the exception of CDC, funding in this figure is based on the amount awarded to fund projects under the agencies' activities from fiscal year 2008 through fiscal year 2011. CDC funded one non-research activity—an awareness campaign—from fiscal years 2008 through 2011 that was focused on autism and other developmental disabilities. The funding amount for CDC in this figure represents all funding for the activity, such as awards and activities conducted internally at the agency, with the exception of research—totaling approximately $1.7 million.

After ACL was created in 2012, management of one autism-related activity was moved from Administration for Children and Families to ACL. Because ACL currently manages the activity, it is attributed to ACL in the figure.

Figure 2. Federal Funds Awarded for Non-Research Autism-Related Activities, Fiscal Years 2008 through 2011.

Most of the autism research funded by the agencies is conducted by scientists at external research organizations—known as extramural research—and funded through mechanisms including grants, contracts, and cooperative agreements. To apply for research funding, an institution submits an application on behalf of a principal investigator—the individual who is responsible and accountable for conducting the research—in response to an agency's funding opportunity announcement.[18] Some announcements are targeted to autism, while others are general funding opportunity announcements that may cover a number of topics, including autism, such as announcements soliciting biomedical research. Lastly, some agencies allow the submission of "unsolicited" or "investigator-initiated" applications.[19] Agencies may also fund intramural research related to autism.

Since the passage of the CAA in 2006, the IACC has issued several reports as a means to coordinate HHS autism activities and monitor federal autism activities, some of which were specifically required by the act, such as the strategic plan. [20] The IACC published its first strategic plan in 2009. The most recent strategic plan was organized into seven questions that correspond to seven research areas. For example, the first question in the strategic plan—"When should I be concerned?"— corresponds to research related to the diagnosis of autism. Each research area contains specific short- and long-term research objectives.[21] Over the years, more have been added, for a total of 78 objectives in the most recent plan.[22] Figure 3 outlines the research areas and number of objectives.

The IACC also produces an annual Autism Spectrum Disorder Research Portfolio Analysis Report, which is organized by the seven research areas of the strategic plan. It includes information on research projects funded by federal and nonfederal entities related to autism, including budget information, for a single fiscal year.[23] The portfolio analysis also categorizes the research projects to the specific objectives in the strategic plan; and indicates if an objective has been fulfilled based on the funding of projects related to that objective in a given year.[24] In order to prepare the portfolio analysis, OARC collects data from federal and nonfederal entities on the autism-related research projects they funded in a certain fiscal year. OARC works with these entities to categorize each project according to the research areas and objectives in the strategic plan. See appendix II for a description of the reports produced by the IACC.

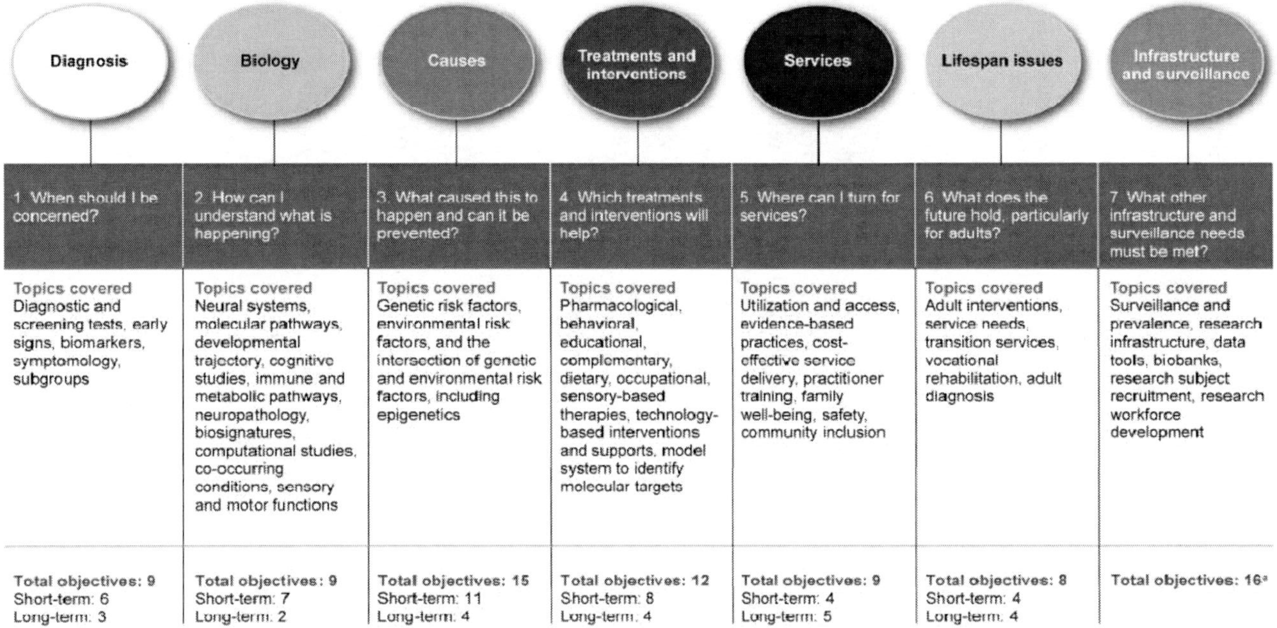

Source: GAO analysis of data from the National Institute of Mental Health, Office of Autism Research Coordination on behalf of the Interagency Autism Coordinating Committee.

Note: According to the IACC, the "topics covered" do not necessarily encompass all projects funded in each research area.

[a]The IACC considers the 16 objectives for the research area, infrastructure and surveillance, to be both short- and long-term objectives.

Figure 3. Interagency Autism Coordinating Committee (IACC) Strategic Plan Research Areas, July 2012.

In July 2012, the IACC released a companion database to its portfolio analysis, referred to as the "IACC/OARC portfolio analysis web tool" (web tool).[25] The web tool contains information on the specific research projects included in the 2008, 2009, and 2010 portfolio analysis reports. For each project in a given fiscal year (i.e., 2008, 2009, or 2010), the web tool displays information, such as funding agency, principal investigator, funded amount, institution, project description, as well as the strategic plan research area and objective associated with the project. For example, users can sort projects by research area—such as diagnosis— and see all projects included in a particular year's portfolio analysis related to that research area.

The CAA requires the IACC to meet twice annually, and it has met, on average, five times a year since 2008.[26] These meetings often include presentations from experts about specific topics related to recent autism research and service activities, federal agency updates, as well as time to discuss general IACC business, such as how committee members want to move forward with specific tasks, including updating the strategic plan. The meetings also include time for public comments. The IACC subcommittees meet more frequently to further discuss activities and carry out related tasks.

For several years, we have reported on the need for the federal government to strive for greater efficiency and effectiveness by eliminating duplication.[27] This is particularity critical when multiple agencies are involved in the same programmatic or policy area, as is the case with autism research and other autism-related activities. Without effective monitoring and sharing of information among federal agencies about planned or funded autism research or other autism-related activities, agencies may use available funds inefficiently due to duplication of effort. Monitoring such research can be done by searching databases, such as Grants.gov and Clinicaltrials.gov, which contain information on federally funded grant programs and clinical research studies, respectively.[28] Also, some agencies have databases that contain information on the grants and activities they have funded, which are available to the public. For example, NIH's Research Portfolio Online Reporting Tools Expenditures and Results (RePORTER) database includes information on the expenditures and results of NIH funded research, including autism research.

In addition, we have reported on the importance of coordination between federal agencies for many years. We have noted that strategic plans can be effective tools to drive agency collaboration and establish complementary goals and strategies for achieving results.[29] Such plans can reinforce accountability for the collaboration by aligning agency goals and strategies with those of the collaborative efforts.

In our prior work we have also established that measuring and reporting progress on collaborative efforts—such as through the use of short- and long-term strategic objectives—is a best practice for interagency collaboration, as well as an important internal control standard for the federal government.[30]

The Majority of Federally-Funded Autism Research Was Potentially Duplicative, while Non-Research Activities Were Not

We found that most of the autism research projects had the potential to be duplicative. The non-research projects did not.

Most of the Autism Research Funded Was Potentially Duplicative

Of the 1,206 research projects funded by federal agencies from fiscal years 2008 through 2012, 84 percent—or 1,018 projects—had the potential to be duplicative.[31] We found that each of the 11 agencies that funded autism research during this period funded at least 1 autism research project in the same strategic plan objective as another agency, creating the potential for duplication.

Additionally, some objectives were funded by multiple agencies. For example, NIH—which funded the majority of autism research projects—funded projects in the same strategic plan objective as most of the other agencies. In many instances, 3 or more agencies funded research projects under the same objective. For example, 5 agencies—AHRQ, DOD, Education, HRSA, and NIH— awarded approximately $15.2 million for 20 autism research projects related to 1 objective. This objective was to test methods to improve dissemination, implementation, and sustainability of evidence-based interventions, services, and supports in diverse community settings. Four agencies—DOD, Education, HRSA, and NIH—awarded approximately $4.1 million for eight autism research projects to develop at least two individualized community-based interventions to improve quality-of-life or health outcomes for the spectrum of adults with autism. See appendix III for the number of agency research projects and funding amounts for each strategic plan objective.

In addition, many research projects, while not categorized to a specific strategic plan objective, were related to the same research area; and, therefore, may be potentially duplicative. For example, 3 agencies—DOD, NIH, and NSF—awarded approximately $173.0 million for 264 projects in the biology research area, but these projects were not related to a specific objective.[32]

In addition to identifying potential duplication among the federally-funded autism research projects, we obtained additional data from HRSA, AHRQ, and Education that allowed us to identify actual duplication in 4 of the research projects funded by these agencies.[33] HRSA and AHRQ both funded systematic reviews of scientific papers looking at examining effective interventions for children and adolescents with autism.[34] According to HRSA officials, 1 of the agency's grantees was charged with developing guidelines on effective autism interventions for children and adolescents. During this process, they examined 101 scientific papers. AHRQ officials contacted HRSA, and although HRSA's project was underway, AHRQ decided to fund 2 research projects: 1 project reviewing evidence from 183 papers on interventions for children, and 1 project reviewing evidence from 32 papers on interventions for adolescents and young adults. Thirty-one of these papers were reviewed by both HRSA's and AHRQ's grantees. Although HRSA's project led to the development of guidelines for interventions on behavioral health of children and adolescents with autism while AHRQ's projects did not, the projects evaluated many of the same studies for the same population. In addition to the HRSA and AHRQ projects, Education funded a project examining an intervention model of applied behavior analysis for children with disabilities, including autism. The 2 studies included in Education's project were also included in 1 of the AHRQ projects.[35]

Most agency officials we spoke with said that they consider the research funded by their agencies to be different than autism research funded by other agencies; however, we found that at least 4 agencies funded autism research in the same research area. The most commonly funded projects were in the area of biology (423 projects), followed by treatment and interventions (253 projects), and causes (159 projects). NIH funded a majority of the autism research projects in 5 of the 7 research areas. See figure 4 for the agencies that funded autism research projects by research area.

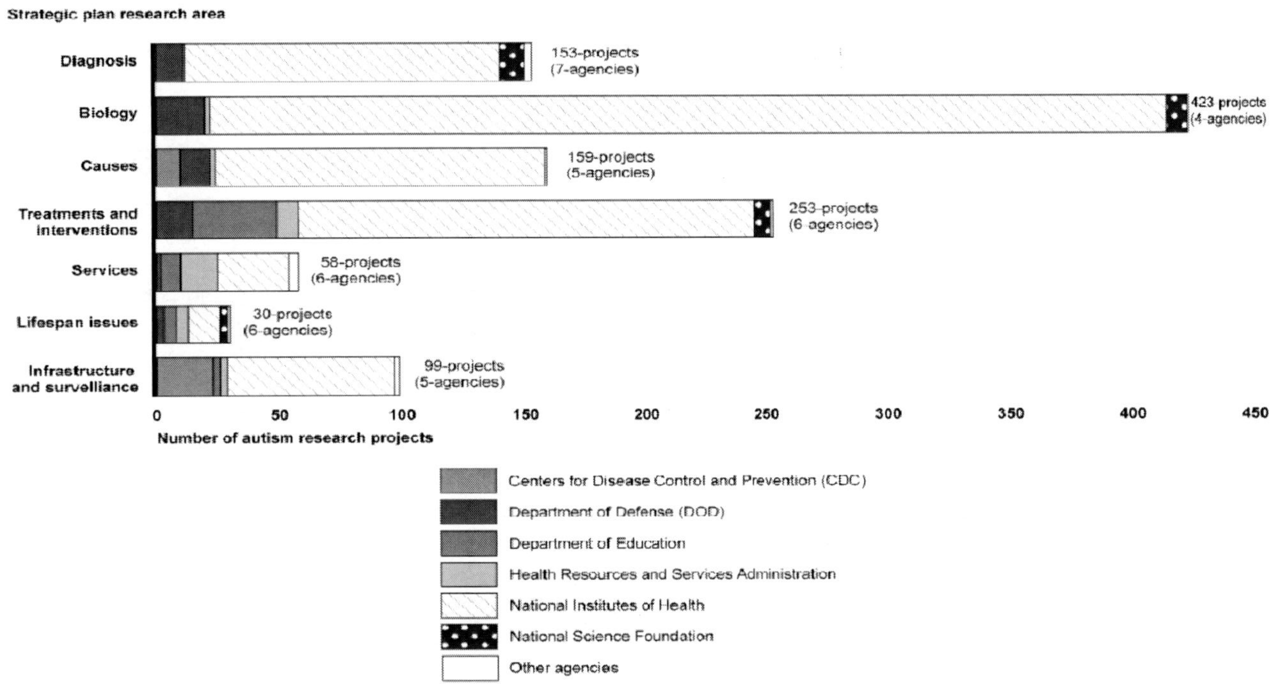

Source: GAO analysis of data from the Interagency Autism Coordinating Committee (IACC) and federal agencies that funded autism research.

Notes: From fiscal years 2008 through 2012, 6 autism projects were included in IACC data, but were categorized as "not specific to any research area," and 16 projects were not included in IACC data and, therefore, not categorized to the research areas. Furthermore, from fiscal years 2008 through 2011, CDC awarded funds for 9 research projects on autism and other developmental disabilities as part of its non-research autism-related activity, *Learn the Signs. Act Early.* CDC categorized the entire activity to the services research area; however, these 9 research projects are not included in the figure because it was unclear if the individual research projects under *Learn the Signs. Act Early.* would also be categorized to the services research area. DOD's research projects include projects funded from DOD's fiscal years 2008 through 2011 appropriations. DOD's fiscal year 2012 appropriation for its medical research programs, including autism, was available for obligation through the end of fiscal year 2013—September 30, 2013. At the time of our review, DOD had not submitted data on its fiscal year 2012 research projects in response to the Office of Autism Research Coordination's request. As a result, the number of autism research projects for DOD does not include DOD's projects for fiscal year 2012.

The agencies included as "other agencies" in each research area are: Administration for Children and Families, Agency for Healthcare Research and Quality (AHRQ), and Substance Abuse and Mental Health Services Administration in diagnosis; Environmental Protection Agency in causes; AHRQ in treatments and interventions; AHRQ and Centers for Medicare & Medicaid Services (CMS) in services; AHRQ in lifespan issues; and CMS in infrastructure and surveillance.

Figure 4. Number of Federal Agencies' Autism Research Projects Funded, by Research Area, Fiscal Years 2008 through 2012.

Non-Research Autism-Related Activities Were Not Duplicative

The five agencies that funded non-research autism-related activities from fiscal years 2008 through 2011—ACL, CDC, DOD, Education, and HRSA—funded activities that were not duplicative.

HRSA and Education both funded training activities related to autism, but we determined that these activities were not duplicative. Among other things, HRSA's training activities train health care professionals, such as pediatric practitioners, residents, and graduate students, to provide evidence-based services to children with autism and other developmental disabilities and their families; and train specialists to provide comprehensive diagnostic evaluations to address the shortage of professionals who can confirm or rule out an autism diagnosis. Education's training activities focus on the education setting; for example, to prepare personnel in special education, related services, early intervention, and regular education to work with children with disabilities, including autism.

Additionally, DOD and ACL both funded a publicly available website to provide information on services available to individuals with autism. However, we determined that these websites were not duplicative. DOD's website was developed for military families to provide them with information on the educational services that are close to specific military installations in select states. The ACL website is broader than the DOD website, focusing on individuals with autism and other developmental disabilities, their families, and other targeted key stakeholders concerned with autism.

We determined that CDC is the only agency funding an awareness campaign on autism and other developmental disabilities. CDC's *Learn the Signs. Act Early.* campaign promotes awareness of healthy developmental milestones in early childhood, the importance of tracking each child's development, and the importance of acting early if there are concerns.[36] This activity also includes an initiative that works with state, territorial, and national partners to improve early childhood systems by enhancing collaborative efforts to improve screening and referral to early intervention services; and to promote *Learn the Signs. Act Early.* messages and tools and improve early identification efforts in their state.

See appendix IV for a list of non-research autism-related activities, as well as the purpose, strategy, and target populations of those activities.

The IACC's and Federal Agencies' Efforts to Coordinate and Monitor Federal Autism Activities Were Limited

We found that the IACC members' views regarding the committee's efforts to coordinate HHS autism activities and monitor federal autism activities were mixed; and the IACC's efforts to coordinate HHS autism activities and monitor federal autism activities were limited by the data the IACC uses. Further, agencies' own efforts to coordinate and monitor autism activities were limited.

Members' Views on IACC Coordination and Monitoring Efforts Were Mixed

Members of the IACC provided mixed views on the usefulness of the IACC's efforts to coordinate HHS autism activities and monitor federal autism activities through its meetings and select documents. Many of the IACC members we spoke with said the IACC meetings aided coordination and monitoring. Specifically, five of the eight federal members—ACL, CDC, CMS, HRSA, and NIH—as well as two of the six nonfederal members we spoke with, stated that the IACC meetings aided coordination and monitoring among HHS and other federal IACC members by providing an opportunity for agencies to learn about others' activities and investments. However, five federal IACC members—AHRQ, CMS, DOD, Education, and HRSA—and one nonfederal member also stated that the information shared during the meetings is typically at a high level and the structure of the meetings provides little opportunity to discuss detailed information. Therefore, it would be difficult to prevent duplication of autism activities through the meetings alone. Education and CMS officials commented that more information sharing would be helpful. A CMS official stated that it would be beneficial for federal agencies to discuss autism activities they are considering funding. However, an Education official stated that while this type of exchange would be beneficial, the official cautioned about the type of information that could be shared in a public setting, such as an IACC meeting. For example, the official stated that providing information to the public on the focus and requirements of a funding opportunity announcement before it is officially released could provide some parties with a competitive advantage and could violate federal regulations. HRSA officials stated that, while specific projects are not usually discussed at meetings, the high-level information shared during meetings is useful; if they need more information they would contact the agency directly. For example, HRSA officials told us that, in one instance, officials from DOD contacted HRSA after hearing about HRSA's autism activities during an IACC meeting. In addition, following an IACC meeting, officials from NIH, CDC, and a nonfederal IACC member organization came together to fund a research project to investigate reports of elevated prevalence of autism among Somali American children in Minneapolis, Minn. Officials from three agencies—CDC, DOD, and NIH—told us that they use the strategic plan and portfolio analysis—which are key documents used by the IACC to coordinate and monitor federal autism activities— when setting priorities for their autism programs and to learn of autism activities conducted by other agencies. For example, NIH officials stated that the specific objectives in the strategic plan allowed them to quickly develop announcements for new projects in fiscal years 2009 and 2010, for which the agency was appropriated additional funds under the American Recovery and Reinvestment Act of 2009. In addition, within DOD, the Office of Congressionally Directed Medical Research Programs' Autism Research Program Integration Panel—an advisory group that reviews autism research applications submitted to DOD—used information from the IACC's strategic plan and portfolio analysis, as well as other sources of information, when determining its autism research priorities.[37]

In contrast, officials from three agencies that are members of the IACC, and two agencies that are not IACC members, but fund autism research, told us that they do not regularly use these IACC documents.[38] Some of the agencies stated that the type of research they fund is different from the type of research identified in the strategic plan. For example, although we found that NSF has funded projects related to autism, officials from NSF—which is not a member of the IACC—said that the agency does not specifically solicit autism research, so they do not consider the strategic plan when selecting research proposals. Education officials also stated that the type of autism-related research the agency funds involves the development and testing of interventions to improve developmental and educational outcomes, which do not fit with the strategic plan objectives. However, we found that the strategic plan did include a research area focused on interventions, as well as one related to lifespan issues—two areas that could encompass the type of autism-related research funded by Education.[39] Education officials also stated that, because the agency provides broad guidance for research applications, much of Education's research is investigator-initiated; therefore, the agency would not be able to direct much research toward the objectives in the strategic plan.

We also found that the IACC may have missed opportunities to coordinate federal autism activities and reduce duplication of effort and resources. Although the CAA requires the IACC to coordinate HHS autism activities and monitor federal autism activities, OARC officials told us that the prevention of duplication among individual projects in agency portfolios is not specified in the CAA as one of the IACC's statutory responsibilities, and therefore, is not a focus of the IACC. OARC officials explained that it is up to individual federal agencies to use the information contained in the IACC's strategic plan and portfolio analysis and the related web tool to prevent duplication. OARC officials acknowledged that the IACC could choose to use the portfolio analysis to make recommendations for increased interagency coordination, but to date this has not occurred. In terms of the role of OARC, OARC officials said they do not review the data that they collect on behalf of the IACC for duplication or for coordination opportunities. Instead, they said that they fulfill their role in assisting the IACC in its cross-agency coordination activities in other ways, such as by facilitating interagency communication and gathering information.

Shortcomings in the IACC's Data Limited Its Ability to Coordinate and Monitor Federal Autism Activities

We found that the data the IACC used and reported in its portfolio analysis and related web tool had limitations that prevented the IACC from effectively monitoring and coordinating federal autism research and non-research activities. Specifically, we found that the data used by the IACC had the following limitations:

- *Outdated information.* The most recent portfolio analysis and web tool contained data from 2010, which was not useful in identifying gaps in current research as they relate to the strategic plan objectives. For example, CDC officials commented that a more up-to-date portfolio analysis would have been helpful when developing the 2012 strategic plan update, which was prepared in the summer and fall of 2012. Additionally, agencies could not use these data to determine whether a prospective autism-related research project was potentially duplicative of a new project funded since 2010.

- *Not tracked over time.* Information on the research projects relating to autism was reported for one year only and not for multiple years combined. The portfolio analysis and web tool included information on whether a certain objective in the strategic plan had been met for a particular year; however, information on the progress of the objectives over time had not been presented.[40] OARC officials stated that the goal of the portfolio analysis and web tool has not been to compare funding year to year.
- *Inconsistent.* The guidance and methodology for determining what projects constitute research has changed over the years. As a result, the projects included in the portfolio analysis and web tool have varied. Specifically, the 2010 portfolio analysis included projects HRSA funded under its training activities—training health professionals on evidenced-based services for those with autism and other developmental disabilities, and how to confirm or rule out an autism diagnosis. According to OARC officials, these projects were not included in prior years because they were not aware that HRSA's training projects could have possible relevance to the objectives in the strategic plan. Once OARC learned about these projects, OARC officials asked HRSA to include these projects in the portfolio analysis. Subsequently, in response to feedback from the IACC, OARC's recent request to agencies for 2011 and 2012 funding data included guidance stating that agencies should not include projects that solely involve the training of professionals.[41]
- *Incomplete.* We identified 16 autism research projects that were not included in the IACC data, such as a DOD Air Force study on autism gene sequencing and other topics, and autism research projects funded by Education and HRSA.[42] For example, Education officials told us that the agency funded a study in 2008 to address challenges faced by geographically remote families in accessing effective intervention services for their young children diagnosed with autism; however, this project was not included in the IACC's data.[43]

Besides autism research projects, the portfolio analysis and strategic plan contain limited information on non-research autism-related activities, and the IACC did not have a mechanism to collect information on such activities. As part of its data collection for the portfolio analysis, the IACC sometimes obtained information from agencies on non-research autism-related activities that related to the strategic plan, which were subsequently included in the portfolio analysis. However, agencies, organizations, and individuals seeking information on non-research autism-related activities would likely not expect to find such information in the portfolio analysis and web tool because the titles and descriptions imply that they are focused on autism research.[44] According to many nonfederal IACC members, as well as some federal members, the IACC has not given enough attention to the coordination and monitoring of non-research autism-related activities. As a result, a complete accounting of federal non-research activities was lacking. These data limitations hindered the IACC's efforts to coordinate HHS autism research and monitor the federal autism environment, as required by the CAA. We have previously reported that tracking and monitoring are key activities that can benefit interagency collaborative mechanisms, such as the IACC. [45] In addition, federal internal control standards state that organizations should monitor and assess their performance over time to help ensure that they meet their goals and objectives. Federal internal control standards also call for data that allows for comparisons and assessments on organizational progress.[46] However, the shortcomings in the IACC's data prevent accurate measurement of its effort to coordinate and monitor. For example, without assessing data over time, information on progress and gaps in autism research may be misleading and incomplete. We found that, when looking across multiple years, some agencies funded more autism research projects than were suggested in the associated strategic plan objective, whereas other objectives were not funded by an agency.[47] In addition, inconsistency in the data made it difficult to accurately determine how much an increase in the funding of autism research was due to an actual increase in research versus the inclusion of more projects in the analysis. For example, in its most recent portfolio analysis, the IACC stated that, while many funders participating in the previous analysis increased their investment levels, the increase in autism research funding, when compared to the prior year's report, was largely attributed to the inclusion of more projects and funders. Lastly, we believe that such shortcomings in the data limited agencies ability to use these data to identify opportunities for coordination of resources or projects, or identify duplicative research that could have been avoided, consolidated, or eliminated. In fiscal year 2013, during the course of our review, the IACC took actions to reduce some of its data limitations. In January 2013, OARC, on behalf of the IACC, began collecting data on the autism research projects agencies funded in 2011 and 2012. OARC officials stated that they were collecting this data in order to have more recent information for the IACC to use when developing the 2013 strategic plan update. In addition, during its July 2013 committee meeting, the IACC discussed its intentions to update the strategic plan, including reviewing more recent agency data, as well as data over time. For the IACC's review, for example, OARC planned to prepare data on agencies' autism research projects funded from 2008 through 2012 for each research area and the objectives within those areas. When we asked whether this dataset would be made publicly available, OARC officials stated that the data would be published around the time the portfolio analysis is published, which OARC expects to be in the first quarter of calendar year 2014.[48] In September 2013, OARC began providing certain IACC members with draft templates for how some of these data could be presented. The committee planned to develop the 2013 update to the strategic plan in the fall of 2013 and expected to complete the report by December 31, 2013.

Federal Agencies' Coordination and Monitoring of Autism Activities Was Limited

We found limited instances of coordination among the 10 agencies that we reviewed and found that all of these agencies lacked robust or routine procedures for monitoring federal autism activities. Two agencies, CDC and HRSA, coordinated their autism activities by holding regular meetings to, for example, share information on project updates and explore potential opportunities for collaboration. These agencies coordinated their autism activities in a manner that was consistent with key collaboration practices to enhance and sustain coordination that we have identified in prior work.[49] These key practices include agreeing on roles and responsibilities and establishing a means to operate across organizational boundaries. For example, officials from CDC and HRSA worked together with HRSA grantees to promote and evaluate CDC's awareness campaign for autism and other developmental disabilities. CDC officials said that they and HRSA officials have a good understanding of each other's roles and autism activities.

A few agencies co-managed individual autism research projects and held joint meetings with their grantees.[50] For example, EPA and NIH jointly funded research studying environmental exposures in relation to children's health and autism. Similarly, CDC and NIH jointly funded a research project to investigate reports of elevated prevalence of autism among Somali-American children in Minneapolis. According to CDC officials, the joint effort allowed CDC to provide scientific oversight and technical assistance to the grantee, which used CDC's surveillance methods, while NIH provided scientific consultation. The two agencies, along with a nonfederal organization, held regular meetings with their grantee. A few agencies also had officials that served on other agencies' advisory committees related to autism research or other autism-related activities. For example, DOD's Autism Research Program Integration Panel included a representative from NIH in fiscal years 2008 and 2009, and recently included a representative from CDC who had been on the panel since fiscal year 2011. In addition, a CDC official served on an advisory council related to research HRSA funded on autism interventions for physical health; and a HRSA official served as a liaison on an advisory board for a non-research autism-related activity funded by Education. Agencies also provided examples of informal communications they had with other agencies. For example, although there were no regularly scheduled formal meetings with NIH, officials from CDC and HRSA stated that their staff have ongoing informal communication with NIH staff and may involve them in grant reviews, workshops, and meetings. CDC and HRSA may also preview NIH funding opportunity announcements. NIH officials told us that, when NIH is considering funding research similar to that of another agency, NIH staff discuss their plans with that agency to pre-empt unnecessarily duplicative research; NIH officials provided one example of a recent instance when they contacted another agency in this regard. However, NIH officials also stated that because many of the agency's research project applications, including those related to autism research, are investigator-initiated, coordination with other agencies during program development is not always possible. Nevertheless, we noted that agencies did not have robust and routine monitoring procedures or methods to ensure that duplication is minimized. As established in our recent duplication work, it is important for agencies that fund research on topics of common interest, such as autism, to monitor each others' activities in order to reduce the potential for unnecessary duplication.[51] It is also a federal internal control standard that agencies establish a means of communicating with, and obtaining information from, other agencies that could impact their operations, performance, and resource allocations.[52] Of the 10 agencies we spoke with, 5 agencies stated that they monitored federal autism activities by searching databases or websites, but those searches were limited and some agencies did not have formal policies or procedures that staff must follow. For example, DOD and NIH conducted searches to ensure that the principal investigator was not receiving funding from another agency for the same project.[53] AHRQ also may conduct a similar search related to the principal investigator. However, these limited searches would not identify whether these agencies were funding similar projects led by different principal investigators. The 5 agencies told us they conducted the following searches:

- AHRQ officials told us that, before funding a systematic review, they reviewed a number of databases, such as RePORTER and www.clinicaltrials.gov, a database that contains information on federally funded as well as non-federally funded studies. AHRQ officials said that they search the databases to determine if a similar systematic review has been conducted or if a major clinical trial is underway. In the latter instance, AHRQ may wait to fund a systematic review until the clinical trial is complete so it can be included in its review. AHRQ officials told us that for those projects that are not systematic reviews, they searched databases using the principal investigator's last name and the term "autism."
- CDC officials stated that they informally review Grants.gov, the central grant identification and application portal for federal grant programs, when developing a new program announcement.
- DOD officials told us that, before funding a project, they search the NIH database RePORTER—which includes projects funded by NIH— using the principal investigator's name and other terms. DOD officials also stated that they review NIH's institutes' websites as a source of information when determining their autism research priorities.
- HRSA officials said that they check RePORTER for similar autism projects on a quarterly basis using the search terms "autism" and "ASD;" however, the agency does not have written policies for the search. HRSA officials told us that they do not search other agencies' websites or databases on a regular basis.
- NIH officials told us that they search their own databases, including a database that contains information about research funded by NIH, AHRQ, CDC, and other agencies.

Several agency officials also told us that they rely on their peer reviewers, other experts, and project officers to have knowledge of the current autism research environment. For example, officials at AHRQ, DOD, Education, and NIH stated that they consider the opinions of peer reviewers, who are typically scientists or professors who review proposals for scientific merit, to determine whether applications may be duplicative of other research. DOD officials also told us that they rely on their Autism Research Program Integration Panel to be knowledgeable of research funded by other agencies. NIH officials stated that project officers have an in-depth understanding of the scientific subject matter related to their grant portfolios.[54] According to NIH officials, their project officers keep abreast of the scientific literature, attend professional and scientific meetings, and interact with the principal investigator and other scientific staff at the grantee institution. Apart from their participation on the IACC, some agencies did not provide examples of actions they had taken to coordinate with or monitor other agencies' autism activities. For example, when we asked about the mechanisms used to coordinate and monitor autism activities, CMS stated that it interacted with other federal agencies through its IACC participation. Officials also stated that it is not common for CMS to fund autism research projects. In addition, although HRSA told us that one of their staff participated on an advisory committee for one Education non-research autism-related activity, Education officials did not provide examples of coordination efforts; Education is a member of the IACC. NSF, which is not an IACC member, does not coordinate or monitor its autism activities with other agencies to prevent unnecessary duplication. NSF officials stated that while they may fund research related to autism, they generally do not solicit autism research. Given that each agency we reviewed funded at least one autism research project in the same strategic plan objective as another agency from fiscal years 2008 through 2012, and some objectives were funded by multiple agencies, current coordination and monitoring efforts may be insufficient. For example, while DOD officials told us that they review NIH websites when determining their autism research priorities, we found that DOD funded autism research projects related to most of the same strategic plan objectives as NIH, which could potentially result in unnecessarily duplicative research.[55] In addition, NSF—an agency that did not coordinate with other agencies regarding autism research—funded research projects that related to the same objectives as projects funded by both NIH and DOD.

CONCLUSION

Funding similar research on the same topic area—such as autism—is sometimes appropriate and necessary; for example, for purposes of replicating or corroborating prior research results. In addition, having multiple agencies with different expertise involved in autism activities— both research and other related activities—can be advantageous. One such advantage is that agencies may be better able to tailor research or other programs to suit their specific missions and needs. However, having multiple agency involvement can also make it challenging to identify gaps and allocate resources across the federal government efficiently. Given that 12 federal agencies spent at least $1.4 billion on autism research and other autism-related activities from fiscal years 2008 through 2012, and that multiple agencies have funded autism research related to the same objectives, it is incumbent on the agencies to effectively coordinate and monitor each other's autism research. Not doing so could lead to numerous projects being funded to address a few specific areas within the realm of autism research—some of the projects having the potential to be unnecessarily duplicative—while other areas may be left unexplored.

Interagency committees—such as the IACC—can aid agencies' efforts to coordinate and monitor. The IACC's charge to coordinate autism activities of HHS and to monitor federal autism activities provides the IACC with the opportunity to play an important role in maximizing the effectiveness and efficiency of the federal investment in autism activities, and in minimizing the inefficient use of federal resources due to unnecessary duplication of effort. However, the weaknesses in the IACC's data limits agencies' abilities to identify the autism research that has been recently funded, any gaps in or potential opportunities for funding, possible opportunities for efficiencies, or possible duplication. In addition, the focus of the strategic plan and portfolio analysis on autism research and limited focus on non-research activities restricts the ability of the IACC to monitor non-research autism-related activities funded by the federal government, and may affect agencies' abilities to identify duplicative efforts related to these activities. Apart from the IACC, there are limited instances of agencies independently coordinating their own autism activities. Agencies lack robust and routine procedures for monitoring the projects that other agencies are funding. Such monitoring would help avoid unnecessary duplication of autism research. It may also help identify potential opportunities for further coordination, since agencies can only coordinate with each other when they are aware of relevant research or other activities. Ultimately, agency coordination and monitoring would help ensure that scarce federal resources are used as efficiently as possible.

RECOMMENDATIONS

To improve the usefulness of IACC data and enhance its efforts to coordinate HHS autism activities and monitor all federally funded autism activities, we recommend that the Secretary of Health and Human Services direct the IACC and NIH, in support of the IACC, to take the following three actions:

- provide consistent guidance to federal agencies when collecting data for the portfolio analysis and web tool so that information can be more easily and accurately compared over multiple years;
- create a document or database that provides information on non-research autism-related activities funded by the federal government and make this document or database publicly available; and
- identify projects through its monitoring of federal autism activities—including OARC's annual collection of data for the portfolio analysis and the IACC's annual process to update the strategic plan—that may result in unnecessary duplication and thus may be candidates for consolidation or elimination, and identify potential coordination opportunities among agencies.

To promote better coordination among federal agencies that fund autism research and avoid the potential for unnecessary duplication before research projects are funded, we recommend that the Secretary of Health and Human Services, the Secretary of Defense, the Secretary of Education, and the Director of NSF each determine methods for identifying and monitoring the autism research conducted by other agencies, including by taking full advantage of monitoring data the IACC develops and makes available.

AGENCY COMMENTS AND OUR EVALUATION

We provided a draft of this report to DOD, Education, HHS, and NSF for comment. Our first recommendation was directed to HHS exclusively. HHS did not concur with this recommendation. Our second recommendation was directed toward all four agencies. DOD agreed with this recommendation. Although the other three agencies did not explicitly state agreement with the recommendation, their comments suggested that they view the opportunity to enhance the coordination of federal autism research activities positively. These three agencies also expressed concern about certain of the report's conclusions as described in detail below. In addition to general comments, Education and HHS also provided technical comments, which we incorporated as appropriate. HHS did not concur with our first recommendation that the agency take three specific actions to improve the usefulness of the IACC data.

First, HHS did not concur that the IACC and NIH should take action to provide consistent guidance to federal agencies when collecting data for the portfolio analysis. HHS commented that OARC has used a consistent methodology and provided consistent guidance to agencies when collecting data for the portfolio analysis on behalf of the IACC. It also emphasized that it has balanced the need for consistency with the need to be responsive to feedback from the IACC and from those participating in the portfolio analysis. While we agree with HHS that it is important to be responsive to feedback and make adjustments to guidance as necessary to improve data collection, we believe that annual changes of the type we observed are not productive. The exclusion of training projects in one year of data collection, their inclusion in the subsequent year, and their partial exclusion in the next year is a change in methodology and guidance that makes it difficult to analyze and interpret data over time. Additionally, OARC did not provide consistent guidance to organizations—both federal and nonfederal—that submit information for inclusion in the portfolio analysis. For example, in the year that OARC requested HRSA to include its training projects in the portfolio analysis, it did not make the same request of other organizations and its guidance did not mention that these specific types of projects should be included in the data submitted to OARC. We therefore continue to believe that guidance should be developed so that accurate, consistent, and meaningful comparisons of changes in federal funding of autism research can be made over time and used to inform future funding decisions. Second, HHS did not concur that the IACC and NIH should take action to create a document or database that provides information on non-research autism-related activities. HHS commented that this information was already publicly accessible and cited a report to Congress published by OARC in December 2010.[56] While this report contained information on federally funded autism activities from fiscal years 2006 through 2009, it did not include all of the non-research autism-related activities we identified in our report. In addition, while helpful, the report is nonetheless a static document. There is no single repository for information on non-research autism-related activities funded by the federal government since 2009—a shortcoming that has prevented effective monitoring of these activities since that year. HHS also commented that, as required by the reauthorization of the CAA, it would be providing a report to Congress to be released to the public in the fall of 2013. HHS stated that this report would include information on research, services, and other non-research autism activities that were supported by federal agencies from fiscal years 2010 through 2012. While this document could be a starting point from which the

IACC could begin to regularly catalog non-research autism-related activities, we believe that having a document or database that contains current information on these activities is an important aspect of fulfilling the IACC's responsibility to monitor all federal autism activities, not just research.

Third, HHS did not concur that, through its monitoring activities, the IACC and HHS should take action to identify projects that may result in unnecessary duplication and thus may be candidates for consolidation or elimination. However, HHS said that it will continue to support the IACC in its activities to coordinate HHS efforts and identify opportunities for cross-agency coordination. HHS stated that an analysis by the IACC to identify duplication would not likely provide the type of information on actual duplication needed by agency officials when making funding decisions. HHS said that even if the IACC further refined its analysis to identify several grants on the same general topic within each research objective as potentially duplicative, this type of information would lack adequate specificity to be useful to agency officials who are involved in the grant award process. We agree that the specific projects identified in the analysis proposed by HHS would need to be reviewed further to identify actual duplication—defined as projects with the same purpose, strategies, and target population that are not necessary to, for example, corroborate or replicate prior research results. However, we believe that the IACC's identification of such projects would be worthwhile as it could effectively lead to their further review by the funding agencies. In addition, HHS commented that it does not believe there is too much federal activity related to autism and that the IACC role should not include identification of autism-related projects for elimination. It should be noted that our report does not state—and should not be interpreted as suggesting—that there is too much federal activity related to autism. We recognize that autism is an important public health concern affecting a large number of people. However, this makes it all the more important that scarce federal resources be used wisely. Prudent stewardship requires a careful assessment of research spending. Many agencies currently devote considerable time to identifying and providing HHS with spending information and HHS invests in this data collection. However, we question the purpose of devoting federal resources to collecting these data, if they are not then used to ensure federal funds are used appropriately. The IACC data can be used to drill down to help identify unnecessary duplication and opportunities to enhance coordination. A thorough review of autism data is particularly important to ensure federal funds are used efficiently and effectively. While, we agree that the IACC does not have the authority to eliminate duplicative projects, it does have the responsibility to make recommendations to the Secretary of Health and Human Services. If unnecessary duplication or opportunities to enhance coordination between HHS agencies were identified, the IACC could make related recommendations that would carry important weight.

DOD concurred with our second recommendation to improve coordination among federal agencies, and comments from Education, HHS, and NSF suggest that these agencies support improving the coordination of federal autism research activities. DOD, Education, and NSF commented that they intend to work with the IACC and other agencies to share information related to autism research. HHS agreed that there should be continued coordination to avoid unnecessary duplication across research projects. However, with the exception of DOD, the agencies included comments suggesting that they were concerned with the report's conclusion that some federal autism research projects had the potential to be duplicative. Specifically, the agencies stated the following:

- Education did not concur with the conclusions that the majority of federally-funded autism research projects had the potential to be duplicative. The agency stated that, because the IACC's strategic plan objectives are broad, projects categorized under the same objective cannot be fairly judged as potentially duplicative without more substantial exposition.
- HHS stated that research funded under the same objective does not necessarily indicate duplication, as the objectives represent broad and complex areas of research.
- NSF stated that the categorization of its projects to, for example, the research area of biology, does not indicate that these projects are duplicative of other agencies' projects about the biology of autism.

We stated in our draft report that our methodology of using the categorization of projects to the same strategic plan objective or research area does not indicate actual duplication; however, we added language to the final report to make this point clearer. We agree that more information on the specific projects funded within each objective would need to be assessed in order to determine actual duplication. However, the fact that research is categorized to the same objectives suggests that there may be duplicative projects being funded. Education, HHS, and NSF did not provide any information throughout the course of our work or in their comments indicating that they had reviewed these projects to ensure that they were not unnecessarily duplicative. In addition, two agencies—HHS and NSF—included comments suggesting that they were concerned about the report's conclusion that the coordination and monitoring of federal autism activities were limited. Specifically,

- HHS did not concur with the conclusion that federal agencies' coordination and monitoring of autism activities was limited. HHS commented that it has extensive policies in place to prevent duplicative projects and that it would continue its procedures for avoiding duplication. HHS stated that an NIH research project applicant is required to indicate the other agencies to which the application has been submitted. In addition, the applicant is required to indicate the financial support received for the project. According to HHS, it is the responsibility of NIH staff to review this information to ensure that NIH is not funding the applicant for the same research project funded by another agency. HHS also cited an NIH database that is used extensively by NIH staff to obtain and manage information related to research project funding decisions.
- NSF also commented on activities it undertakes to avoid duplication and stated that it takes steps to ensure that it does not fund the same research project by the same applicant if it is already supported by another agency.

The procedures described by both agencies were outlined in our draft report. While important, they are not sufficiently comprehensive and are limited in that they only look to identify duplicative projects led by the same principle investigator. They do not identify project applications led by another principle investigator that may be unnecessarily duplicative of a project that has already been federally funded—a project with the same purpose, strategies, and target population that is not necessary to, for example, corroborate or replicate prior research results. For example, while the NIH database cited in HHS's comments could be a helpful coordination tool, our report points out that NIH's database search was limited in that its purpose was to ensure that a principal investigator was not receiving funding from another agency for the same project. The search would not identify similar projects led by different principal investigators. Therefore, we stand by our conclusion that these agencies' methods to monitor and coordinate autism activities are limited. HHS also commented that our draft report implied that it is wasteful for more than one federal agency to address a strategic plan objective. HHS said that the strategic plan objectives describe the minimum effort that would be required to address the complex issues set in each objective. Our report does not state this, nor do we believe that having more than one project per objective is inappropriate. Our report acknowledges that funding similar research on the same topic is sometimes appropriate and necessary. We agree that it may be beneficial to have multiple projects and agencies associated with the same strategic plan objective; however, we contend that it is important to carefully review the data to ensure that projects are indeed essential to achieve research goals and not unnecessarily duplicative. Using the data collected by HHS and analyzing it over time, provides an important opportunity for the IACC to determine whether its coordination efforts are successful. Doing so can provide important information on both progress and gaps in autism research, and identify areas of potential duplication to investigate further. For example, as we noted in our draft report, we found that 1 objective—which recommended testing 4 methods to improve dissemination, implementation, and sustainability of evidenced-based interventions, services, and supports in diverse community settings—had 20 projects associated with it that were funded by 5 different agencies from fiscal years 2008 through 2012. We believe it is important that these projects be reviewed further. While all of these projects are perhaps necessary to achieve research goals and are not duplicative, without conducting a thorough review of the data, it is not clear that this is, indeed, the case. Finally, HHS stated that our draft report was incorrect in stating that we had identified 16 projects that were omitted from the IACC's data. HHS said that the number we reported should have been 14. We disagree. We provided OARC with a list of 18 projects that we initially identified as missing from the IACC's data. OARC provided us with additional information for 2 of these projects. As a result, there were 16 projects— with total award funding of approximately $74 million—that we identified that were not included in the IACC's data. Further, HHS explained that the projects that were not included in the IACC data were either projects that the agencies funded before the agencies had been included in the portfolio analysis, or projects that agencies did not submit to OARC during data collection for the portfolio analysis. We understand that, to a certain extent, OARC must rely on federal agencies to disclose the autism research projects they fund. However, 7 of these 16 projects—which were awarded funds totaling approximately $69 million—were NIH-funded projects, the agency in which OARC resides.

Marcia Crosse
Director, Health Care

APPENDIX I: METHODOLOGY FOR ANALYZING POTENTIAL DUPLICATION OF FEDERALLY FUNDED AUTISM RESEARCH AND OTHER ACTIVITIES

Identifying Autism Research Projects and Other Autism-Related Activities

First, we identified federal agencies that funded autism research and other autism-related activities from fiscal years 2008 through 2011 by interviewing the federal agencies on the Interagency Autism Coordinating Committee (IACC) and select nonfederal IACC members; reviewing IACC and agency documentation describing federal autism activities; and searching Grants.gov and the Catalog of Federal Domestic Assistance.[1] We also included any agencies and the related research projects they awarded in fiscal year 2012, as identified in data that agencies submitted to the IACC.

We considered a federal agency to have funded autism research or an autism-related activity if the research project or activity was autism-specific or had an autism-specific component and was supported by federal funds awarded through mechanisms such as grants, cooperative agreements, or contracts, or was research conducted by scientists in government laboratories, known as intramural research. 2 We excluded activities that provided a direct benefit to individuals with autism, such as insurance coverage to specific populations; housing assistance; and supplemental income. We also excluded funding provided to states to offer direct services to individuals with autism or their families, such as educational services. Additionally, we excluded federally funded workshops and meetings from our review. Furthermore, with the exception of intramural research, we excluded activities that the agencies undertook directly. These included, for example, the inclusion of information on an agency website or fact sheets. Finally, we excluded research projects and non-research autism-related activities funded by nonfederal organizations. Based on our analysis, 12 agencies funded autism research and other autism-related activities between fiscal years 2008 and 2012 that met our criteria.

We collected and reviewed the project information from each agency, such as research project numbers, award amounts, and project titles, where applicable, for fiscal years 2008 through 2011.[3,4] We compared the agencies' research projects to the projects in the IACC's Autism Spectrum Disorder Portfolio Analysis Report and web tool data for fiscal years 2008, 2009, and 2010—the most recent portfolio analyses available at the time of our review—

and reconciled any differences with the agencies.[5] In January 2013, while our work was in progress, we learned that the Office of Autism Research Coordination (OARC), on behalf of the IACC, requested fiscal years 2011 and 2012 autism research project data from the agencies for its forthcoming portfolio analysis and web tool, which we obtained from each agency to include in our analysis.[6] We were unable to obtain fiscal year 2012 data for the Department of Defense (DOD). DOD's fiscal year 2012 appropriation for its medical research programs, including autism, was available for obligation through the end of fiscal year 2013—September 30, 2013. At the time of our review, DOD had not submitted data on its fiscal year 2012 research projects in response to OARC's request. As a result, our report does not include data on DOD's fiscal year 2012 autism research.

The research projects and related award amounts included in our review differ from the research projects and funding amounts included in the portfolio analysis and web tool for several reasons:

- The portfolio analysis and web tool included projects funded by nonfederal organizations, which we did not include in our review.
- The portfolio analysis and web tool included research using broader criteria than that used in our review. For example, projects that focused on developmental disabilities in general may have been included in the portfolio analysis even if they did not have a component specific to autism. In addition, the portfolio analysis and web tool included some projects that we did not consider to be research, based on information collected and discussions with the agencies.[7]
- The portfolio analysis and web tool reported projects differently than what we used in our methodology. For example, a project was included twice in the portfolio analysis and web tool if the project received a supplemental award and base funding in the same year. In our analysis, we added the award amounts and counted the project once.[8]
- We identified more research projects than those included in the portfolio analysis web tool.

Determining Potential Duplication of Autism Research Projects

We analyzed potential duplication using the portfolio analysis data, which categorized each project to the research areas and objectives in the IACC's Strategic Plan for Autism Spectrum Disorder Research.[9] Objectives have been added to the strategic plan since its first issuance in 2009. For projects that span multiple years, we used the most recent year's strategic plan research area and objective categories.[10] To determine potential duplication in autism research, we identified research projects that were categorized to the same strategic plan objectives. For those projects that were not categorized to a specific objective, but were categorized to one of the seven research areas, we assessed duplication based on whether they were categorized to the same research area. Determining that projects were categorized to the same strategic plan objective or research area suggests potential, but not actual duplication. Funding similar research on the same topic is sometimes appropriate and necessary; for example, for purposes of replicating or corroborating prior research results. Determining actual duplication for research projects would require a more extensive review of voluminous and scientific data, and was beyond the scope of this study.

Determining Duplication of Non-Research Autism-Related Activities

To assess whether there was actual duplication of non-research autism-related activities we used the framework we established in our previous work, which states that duplication occurs when two or more agencies fund the same activities that target the same users.[11] To determine if the activities were the same, we reviewed each activity's purpose and strategy for achieving that purpose and reviewed the targeted population of the activities.

Data Reliability Assessment

We took several steps to ensure that the data used to produce this report were sufficiently reliable. In addition to comparing agency data to data collected by OARC and following up with agency officials regarding any discrepancies in the data, we also gathered information from agencies on the internal controls they use for maintaining their data. We determined that the data were sufficiently reliable for the purposes of our study.

APPENDIX II: LIST OF INTERAGENCY AUTISM COORDINATING COMMITTEE (IACC) REPORTS

Report	Description
Strategic Plan for Autism Spectrum Disorder Research (2009, 2010, 2011, 2012)	According to the IACC, the Strategic Plan provides a blueprint for autism research that is advisory to the Department of Health and Human Services and serves as a basis for partnerships with other agencies and private organizations involved in autism research and services. The Strategic Plan is organized around seven questions asked by individuals with autism and their families (such as "When should I be concerned?"). Each of the seven sections includes a description of what is generally known from autism research for that particular question and what gaps remain, followed by what was learned during the previous year. The report also sets up short- and long-term research objectives based on autism research opportunities. The Combating Autism Act of 2006 (CAA) requires that the Strategic Plan be updated on an annual basis.
Autism Spectrum Disorder Research Portfolio Analysis Report (2008, 2009, 2010)[a]	The Portfolio Analysis features autism project and funding information for certain federal agencies and private organizations. According to officials within the National Institutes of Health's Office of Autism Research Coordination (OARC), the agencies and organizations in these reports have been identified by the IACC and OARC as being involved in autism research and have agreed to participate.
	According to the IACC, the intent of these analysis reports is to better inform the IACC and interested stakeholders about the funding landscape for a particular year. Additionally, the analysis examines the extent to which a particular year's funding and research topics align with the IACC's most recent Strategic Plan. The IACC reports that the Portfolio Analysis may also be used by federal agencies and private research organizations to help guide future funding priorities by outlining current gaps and opportunities in autism research, as well as serving to highlight current activities and research progress.
Summary of Advances in Autism Spectrum Disorder Research (2007, 2008, 2009, 2010, 2011, 2012)	Each year the IACC releases its list of scientific advances in autism research. As reported by the IACC, the report highlights studies on autism published in the previous year in peer-reviewed journals and selected by members of the IACC. The number of studies featured over the years ranges from 20 to 54. The CAA requires that the IACC produce the Summary of Advances annually.
Autism Spectrum Disorder Research Publications Analysis: The Global Landscape of Autism Research[b]	As reported by the IACC, this report describes several key aspects of worldwide autism research publications, which may be used to inform planning and strategic funding decisions for future autism research. Autism-related research articles published between 1980 and 2010 were analyzed to identify historical trends and publication outputs across the seven questions and research areas of the 2011

Report	Description
	IACC Strategic Plan. Information found in the research publications was also used to assess the institutions conducting autism research, funding organizations supporting the research publications, and the extent of collaboration between authors from different countries and research institutions. Additionally, measures, such as citation counts, were used as an assessment of the impact of the published research. OARC officials told us that there are no plans to update this report annually.

Source: GAO review of IACC documents.

Note: The years listed next to the report title are the years to which the report applies, which may not be the same year the report was published. For example, the 2010 Autism Spectrum Disorder Research Portfolio Analysis Report was published in July 2012.

[a]OARC, National Institute of Mental Health, prepared this report on behalf of the IACC. For the 2009 report, OARC, National Institute of Mental Health, and Acclaro Research Solutions, Inc., prepared the report on behalf of the IACC.

[b]OARC, National Institute of Mental Health, and Thomson Reuters, Inc. prepared this report on behalf of the IACC.

APPENDIX III: FEDERAL AUTISM RESEARCH PROJECTS BY INTERAGENCY AUTISM COORDINATING COMMITTEE STRATEGIC PLAN OBJECTIVE

Eleven federal agencies awarded approximately $1.2 billion to fund autism research projects from fiscal years 2008 through 2012.[1] These agencies are Department of Defense (DOD); Department of Education (Education); the Environmental Protection Agency (EPA); the National Science Foundation (NSF); and 7 agencies within the Department of Health and Human Services—Administration for Children and Families (ACF), Agency for Healthcare Research and Quality (AHRQ), Centers for Disease Control and Prevention (CDC), Centers for Medicare & Medicaid Services (CMS), Health Resources and Services Administration (HRSA), National Institutes of Health (NIH), and Substance Abuse and Mental Health Services Administration (SAMHSA). This appendix includes the autism research projects funded by these agencies, as categorized to the Interagency Autism Coordinating Committee's (IACC) strategic plan objectives. Research projects were categorized to the objective that best describes each project according to the strategic plan; however, research projects may not address all aspects of the objective.

Table 1. Number of Federal Agency Autism Research Projects and Funding by Interagency Autism Coordinating Committee Strategic Plan Objective, by Agency, Fiscal Years 2008 through 2012

Strategic Plan Research Area and Objectives[a]	Description of Objective	Agency	Number of Research Projects	Funds Awarded
Research area 1: Diagnosis				
1.S.A	Develop, with existing tools, at least one efficient diagnostic instrument (i.e., briefer, less time intensive) that is valid in diverse populations for use in large-scale studies by 2011.	NIH	11	$12,863,563
1.S.B	Validate and improve the sensitivity and specificity of new or existing screening and diagnostic tools, including comparative studies of general developmental screening versus autism-specific screening tools, in both high-risk and population-based samples, including those from resource-poor international settings and those that are diverse in terms of age, socio-economic status, race, ethnicity, gender, characteristics of autism, and general level of functioning by 2012.	ACF	1	100,000
		AHRQ	1	1,901,626
		NIH	7	4,620,220
1.S.C	Conduct at least three studies to identify reasons for the health disparities in accessing early screening and diagnosis services, including identification of barriers to implementation of and access to screening, diagnosis, referral, and early intervention services among diverse populations, as defined by socioeconomic status, race, ethnicity, and gender of the child, by 2012.	NIH	2	455,081
		SAMHSA	1	450,000

Strategic Plan Research Area and Objectives[a]	Description of Objective	Agency	Number of Research Projects	Funds Awarded
1.S.D	Conduct at least two studies to understand the impact of early diagnosis on choice of intervention and outcomes by 2015.		No federal projects funded	
1.S.E	Conduct at least one study to determine the positive predictive value and clinical utility (e.g., prediction of co-occurring conditions, family planning) of chromosomal microarray genetic testing for detecting genetic diagnoses for autism in a clinical setting by 2012.	NIH	4	5,282,439
1.S.F	Convene a workshop to examine the ethical, legal, and social implications of autism research by 2011. The workshop should define possible approaches for conducting future studies of ethical, legal, and social implications of autism research, taking into consideration how these types of issues have been approached in related medical conditions.		No federal projects funded	
1.L.A	Identify behavioral and biological markers that separately, or in combination, accurately identify, before age 2, 1 or more subtypes of children at risk for developing autism, and evaluate whether these risk markers or profiles can improve early identification through heightened developmental monitoring and screening by 2014.	DOD	7	3,401,458
		NIH	34	38,116,800
1.L.B	Develop at least five measures of behavioral and/or biological heterogeneity in children or adults with autism, beyond variation in intellectual disability, that clearly relate to etiology and risk, treatment response, and/or outcome by 2015.	DOD	2	694,989
		NIH	35	39,065,410
		NSF	9	8,602,000

Table 1. (Continued)

Strategic Plan Research Area and Objectives[a]	Description of Objective	Agency	Number of Research Projects	Funds Awarded
1.L.C	Identify and develop measures to assess at least three "continuous dimensions" (e.g., social reciprocity, communication disorders, and repetitive/restrictive behaviors) of autism symptoms and severity that can be used by practitioners and/or families to assess response to intervention for people with autism across the lifespan by 2016.	DOD	1	615,000
		NIH	13	11,921,270
1.Other	Not specific to any objective within research area 1.	DOD	1	546,577
		Education	1	1,971,978
		NIH	22	14,291,166
		NSF	1	14,510
Research area 2: Biology				
2.S.A	Support at least four research projects to identify mechanisms of fever, metabolic and/or immune system interactions with the central nervous system that may influence autism during prenatal-postnatal life by 2010.	DOD	2	615,787
		HRSA	1	294,904
		NIH	18	8,873,917
2.S.B	Launch three studies that specifically focus on the neurodevelopment of females with autism, spanning basic to clinical research on sex differences by 2011.	NIH	5	5,320,506
2.S.C	Identify ways to increase awareness among the autism spectrum community of the potential value of brain and tissue donation to further basic research by 2011.		No federal projects funded	

Strategic Plan Research Area and Objectives[a]	Description of Objective	Agency	Number of Research Projects	Funds Awarded
2.S.D	Launch three studies that target improved understanding of the underlying biological pathways of genetic conditions related to autism (e.g., fragile X, Rett syndrome, tuberous sclerosis complex) and how these conditions inform risk assessment and individualized intervention by 2012.	DOD	2	269,444
		NIH	70	46,269,699
2.S.E	Launch three studies that target the underlying biological mechanisms of co-occurring conditions with autism, including seizures/epilepsy, sleep disorders, wandering/elopement behavior, and familial autoimmune disorders, by 2012.	DOD	5	633,738
		HRSA	1	412,872
		NIH	12	16,788,241
2.S.F	Launch two studies that focus on prospective characterization of children with reported regression to investigate potential risk factors by 2012.	NIH	1	1,612,511
2.S.G	Support five studies that associate specific genotypes with functional or structural phenotypes, including behavioral and medical phenotypes (e.g., nonverbal individuals with autism and those with cognitive impairments) by 2015.	DOD	2	663,751
		NIH	25	29,749,080
		NSF	1	276,000
2.L.A	Complete a large-scale, multidisciplinary, collaborative project that longitudinally and comprehensively examines how the biological, clinical, and developmental profiles of individuals, with a special emphasis on females, youths, and adults with autism, change over time as compared to typically developing people by 2020.	NIH	8	24,365,831

Table 1. (Continued)

Strategic Plan Research Area and Objectives[a]	Description of Objective	Agency	Number of Research Projects	Funds Awarded
2.L.B	Launch at least three studies that evaluate the applicability of autism phenotype and/or biological signature findings for performing diagnosis, risk assessment, or clinical intervention by 2015.	NIH	6	2,379,375
2.Other	Not specific to any objective within research area 2.	DOD	9	2,614,769
		NIH	247	167,289,408
		NSF	8	3,097,145
Research area 3: Causes				
3.S.A	Coordinate and implement the inclusion of approximately 20,000 subjects for genome-wide association studies, as well as a sample of 1,200 for sequencing studies to examine more than 50 candidate genes by 2011. Studies should investigate factors contributing to phenotypic variation across individuals who share an identified genetic variant and stratify subjects according to behavioral, cognitive, and clinical features.	NIH	18	37,608,106
3.S.B	Within the highest-priority categories of exposures for autism, identify and standardize at least three measures for identifying markers of environmental exposure in biospecimens by 2011.	NIH	2	116,367
3.S.C	Initiate efforts to expand existing large case-control and other studies to enhance capabilities for targeted gene-environment research by 2011.	EPA	1	2,271,501
		NIH	7	19,628,501
3.S.D	Enhance existing case-control studies to enroll racially and ethnically diverse populations affected by autism by 2011.	NIH	2	188,455

Strategic Plan Research Area and Objectives[a]	Description of Objective	Agency	Number of Research Projects	Funds Awarded
3.S.E	Support at least two studies to determine if there are subpopulations that are more susceptible to environmental exposures (e.g., immune challenges related to infections, vaccinations, or underlying autoimmune problems) by 2012.	NIH	4	1,027,991
3.S.F	Initiate studies on at least 10 environmental factors identified in the recommendations from the 2007 Institute of Medicine report "Autism and the Environment: Challenges and Opportunities for Research" as potential causes of autism by 2012.	CDC	2	846,247
		DOD	2	227,360
		NIH	3	2,423,008
3.S.G	Convene a workshop that explores the usefulness of bioinformatic approaches to identify environmental risks for autism by 2011.		No federal projects funded	
3.S.H	Support at least three studies of special populations or use existing databases to inform our understanding of environmental risk factors for autism in pregnancy and the early postnatal period by 2012. Such studies could include: comparisons of populations differing in geography, gender, ethnic background, exposure history (e.g., prematurity, maternal infection, nutritional deficiencies, toxins), and migration patterns; and comparisons of phenotype (e.g., cytokine profiles), in children with and without a history of autistic regression, adverse events following immunization (such as fever and seizures), and mitochondrial impairment. These studies may also include comparisons of phenotype between children with regressive autism and their siblings.	CDC	1	1,950,669
		DOD	1	143,162
		HRSA	1	383,243
		NIH	4	9,065,939

Table 1. (Continued)

Strategic Plan Research Area and Objectives[a]	Description of Objective	Agency	Number of Research Projects	Funds Awarded
	Emphasis on environmental factors that influence prenatal and early postnatal development is particularly of high priority. Epidemiological studies should pay special attention to include racially and ethnically diverse populations.			
3.S.I	Support at least two studies that examine potential differences in the microbiome of individuals with autism versus comparison groups by 2012.	DOD	1	132,750
3.S.J	Support at least three studies that focus on the role of epigenetics in the etiology of autism, including studies that include assays to measure DNA methylations and histone modifications, and those exploring how exposures may act on maternal or paternal genomes via epigenetic mechanisms to alter gene expression, by 2012.	DOD	4	1,446,871
		NIH	12	17,650,924
3.S.K	Support two studies and a workshop that facilitate the development of vertebrate and invertebrate model systems for the exploration of environmental risks and their interaction with gender and genetic susceptibilities for autism by 2012.	NIH	2	1,582,038
3.L.A	Conduct a multi-site study of the subsequent pregnancies of 1,000 women with a child with autism to assess the impact of environmental factors in a period most relevant to the progression of autism by 2014.	NIH	1	15,154,483
3.L.B	Identify genetic risk factors in at least 50 percent of people with autism by 2014.	DOD	1	142,113
		NIH	47	49,834,683

Strategic Plan Research Area and Objectives[a]	Description of Objective	Agency	Number of Research Projects	Funds Awarded
3.L.C	Determine the effect of at least five environmental factors on the risk for subtypes of autism in the prenatal and early postnatal period of development by 2015.	NIH	4	1,715,618
3.L.D	Support ancillary studies within one or more large-scale, population-based surveillance and epidemiological studies, including U.S. populations, to collect data on environmental factors during preconception, and during prenatal and early postnatal development, as well as genetic data, that could be pooled (as needed) to analyze targets for potential gene/environment interactions by 2015.	CDC	7	39,560,462
		NIH	11	24,271,103
3.Other	Not specific to any objective within research area 3.	DOD	3	328,091
		HRSA	1	99,235
		NIH	17	7,301,273
Research area 4: Treatments and interventions				
4.S.A	Support at least three randomized controlled trials that address co-occurring medical conditions associated with autism by 2010.	HRSA	1	12,724,207
		NIH	3	906,662
4.S.B	Standardize and validate at least 20 model systems (e.g., cellular and/or animal) that replicate features of autism and will allow identification of specific molecular targets or neural circuits amenable to existing or new interventions by 2012.	DOD	10	3,490,339
		NIH	71	64,969,825
4.S.C	Test safety and efficacy of at least five widely used interventions (e.g., nutrition, medications, assisted technologies, sensory integration, medical procedures) that have not been rigorously studied for use in autism by 2012.	DOD	2	1,967,113
		NIH	8	3,008,201

Table 1. (Continued)

Strategic Plan Research Area and Objectives[a]	Description of Objective	Agency	Number of Research Projects	Funds Awarded
4.S.D	Complete two multi-site randomized controlled trials of comprehensive early intervention that address core symptoms, family functioning and community involvement by 2013.	Education	3	3,849,576
		HRSA	1	9,324,929
		NIH	8	22,409,176
4.S.E	Convene a workshop to advance the understanding of clinical subtypes and treatment personalization (i.e., what are the core symptoms to target for treatment studies) by 2011.		No federal projects funded	
4.S.F	Launch randomized controlled trials of interventions, including biological signatures and other measures to predict response, and monitor quality of life and functional outcomes in each of the following groups: Five trials in infants and toddlers by 2013. Three trials in school-aged children and/or adolescents by 2013. Three trials in adults by 2014.	DOD	2	1,905,130
		HRSA	1	564,816
		NIH	18	22,593,856
		NSF	2	585,833
4.S.G	Support at least five studies on interventions for nonverbal individuals with autism by 2012. Such studies may include: projects examining service-provision models that enhance access to augmentative and alternative communication supports in both classroom and adult service-provision settings, such as residential service-provision and the impact of such access on quality of life, communication, and behavior; studies of novel treatment approaches that facilitate communication skills in individuals who are nonverbal, including the components of effective augmentative and alternative communication approaches for specific subpopulations of people with autism;	Education	1	594,514
		NIH	10	8,085,134

Strategic Plan Research Area and Objectives[a]	Description of Objective	Agency	Number of Research Projects	Funds Awarded
	and studies assessing access and use of augmentative and alternative communication for children and adults with autism who have limited or partially limited speech and the impact on functional outcomes and quality of life.			
4.S.H	Support at least two studies that focus on research on health promotion and prevention of secondary conditions in people with autism by 2012. Secondary conditions of interest include weight issues and obesity, injury, and co-occurring psychiatric and medical conditions.	NIH	2	1,324,994
4.L.A	Complete at least three randomized controlled trials on medications targeting core symptoms in people with autism of all ages by 2014.	HRSA	1	571,147
		NIH	13	8,222,554
4.L.B	Develop interventions for siblings of people with autism with the goal of reducing the risk of recurrence by at least 30 percent by 2014.	NIH	3	890,088
4.L.C	Conduct at least one study to evaluate the safety and effectiveness of medications commonly used in the treatment of co-occurring conditions or specific behavioral issues in people with autism by 2015.	DOD	1	588,750
		NIH	9	6,517,612
4.L.D	Support at least five community-based studies that assess the effectiveness of interventions and services in broader community settings by 2015. Such studies may include comparative effectiveness research studies that assess the relative effectiveness of: different and/or combined medical,	Education	22	28,852,321
		HRSA	3	1,635,606
		NIH	9	5,676,567

Table 1. (Continued)

Strategic Plan Research Area and Objectives[a]	Description of Objective	Agency	Number of Research Projects	Funds Awarded
	pharmacological, nutritional, behavioral, service-provision, and parent- or caregiver-implemented treatments; scalable early intervention programs for implementation in underserved, low-resource, and low-literacy populations; and studies of widely used community intervention models for which extensive published data are not available. Outcome measures should include assessment of potential harm as a result of autism treatments, as well as positive outcomes.			
4.Other	Not specific to any objective within research area 4.	AHRQ	1	575,000
		Education	8	3,196,869
		HRSA	2	912,968
		NIH	33	21,515,583
		NSF	5	1,656,731
Research area 5: Services				
5.S.A	Support two studies that assess how variations in and access to services affect family functioning in diverse populations, including underserved populations, by 2012.	HRSA	7	2,295,114
		NIH	5	4,329,526
5.S.B	Conduct one study to examine how self-directed community-based services and supports impact children, youth, and adults with autism across the spectrum by 2014.	HRSA	1	625,994

Strategic Plan Research Area and Objectives[a]	Description of Objective	Agency	Number of Research Projects	Funds Awarded
5.S.C	Implement and evaluate five models of policy and practice-level coordination among state and local agencies to provide integrated and comprehensive community-based supports and services that enhance access to services and supports, self-determination, economic self-sufficiency, and quality of life for people with autism across the spectrum and their families, (which may include access to augmentative and alternative communication technology), with at least one project aimed at the needs of transitioning youth, and at least one study to evaluate a model of policy and practice-level coordination among state and local mental health agencies serving people with autism, by 2015.	CMS	1	198,348
		HRSA	2	1,500,000
5.S.D	Support two studies to examine health, safety, and mortality issues for people with autism by 2012.		No federal projects funded	
5.L.A	Test four methods to improve dissemination, implementation, and sustainability of evidence-based interventions, services, and supports in diverse community settings by 2013.	AHRQ	1	1,486,234
		DOD	2	2,043,525
		Education	3	1,399,235
		HRSA	4	3,179,367
		NIH	10	7,090,682
5.L.B	Test the efficacy and cost-effectiveness of at least four evidence-based services and supports for people with autism across the spectrum and of all ages living in community settings by 2015.	Education	1	499,995

Table 1. (Continued)

Strategic Plan Research Area and Objectives[a]	Description of Objective	Agency	Number of Research Projects	Funds Awarded
5.L.C	Evaluate new and existing pre-service and in-service training to increase skill levels in service providers, including direct support workers, parents and legal guardians, education staff, and public service workers, to benefit the spectrum of people with autism and to promote interdisciplinary practice by 2015.	NIH	3	2,245,210
5.L.D	Evaluate at least two strategies or programs to increase the health and safety of people with autism that simultaneously consider principles of self-determination and personal autonomy by 2015.	Education	1	592,007
		NIH	1	59,998
5.L.E	Support three studies of dental health issues for people with autism by 2015. This should include: one study on the cost-benefit of providing comprehensive dental services, including routine, non-emergency medical and surgical dental services, denture coverage, and sedation dentistry to adults with autism as compared to emergency and/or no treatment; one study focusing on the provision of accessible, person-centered, equitable, effective, safe, and efficient dental services to people with autism; one study evaluating pre-service and in-service training programs to increase skill levels in oral health professionals to benefit people with autism and promote interdisciplinary practice.	NIH	3	915,605

Strategic Plan Research Area and Objectives[a]	Description of Objective	Agency	Number of Research Projects	Funds Awarded
5.Other	Not specific to any objective within research area 5.	AHRQ	1	2,400,000
		CMS	1	145,007
		Education	3	1,444,552
		HRSA	1	793,013
		NIH	7	4,192,955
Research area 6: Lifespan issues				
6.S.A	Launch at least two studies to assess and characterize variation in the quality of life for adults on the autism spectrum as it relates to characteristics of the service delivery system (e.g., safety, integrated employment, post-secondary educational opportunities, community inclusion, self-determination, relationships, and access to health services and community-based services), and determine best practices by 2012.	HRSA	2	700,000
		NIH	3	892,536
		NSF	1	217,996
6.S.B	Evaluate at least one model, at the state and local level, in which existing programs to assist people with disabilities (e.g., Social Security Administration, Rehabilitation Services Administration) meet the needs of transitioning youth and adults with autism by 2013.	Education	2	3,500,000
6.S.C	Develop one method to identify adults across the autism spectrum who may not be diagnosed, or are misdiagnosed, to support service linkage, better understand prevalence, and track outcomes with consideration of ethical issues (insurance, employment, stigma) by 2015.		No federal projects funded	

Table 1. (Continued)

Strategic Plan Research Area and Objectives[a]	Description of Objective	Agency	Number of Research Projects	Funds Awarded
6.S.D	Conduct at least one study to measure and improve the quality of lifelong supports being delivered in community settings to adults across the spectrum with autism through provision of specialized training for direct care staff, parents, and legal guardians, including assessment and development of autism-specific training, if necessary, by 2015.	NIH	1	749,919
6.L.A	Develop at least two individualized community-based interventions that improve quality-of-life or health outcomes for the spectrum of adults with autism by 2015.	DOD	3	713,298
		Education	1	75,000
		HRSA	1	835,499
		NIH	3	2,496,347
6.L.B	Conduct one study that builds on carefully characterized cohorts of children and youth with autism to determine how interventions, services, and supports delivered during childhood impact adult health and quality of life outcomes by 2015.	NIH	3	5,468,332
6.L.C	Conduct comparative effectiveness research that includes a cost-effectiveness component to examine community-based interventions, services, and supports to improve health outcomes and quality of life for adults on the autism spectrum over age 21 by 2018. Topics should include: community housing for people with autism; successful life transitions for people with autism, including from post-secondary education to adult services, employment, sibling relationships, and day programs; and meeting the service and support needs of older adults with autism.	HRSA	1	793,024
		NIH	1	772,496

Strategic Plan Research Area and Objectives[a]	Description of Objective	Agency	Number of Research Projects	Funds Awarded
6.L.D	Conduct implementation research to test the results from comparative effectiveness research in real-world settings, including a cost-effectiveness component to improve health outcomes and quality of life for adults over 21 on the autism spectrum by 2023.		No federal projects funded	
6.Other	Not specific to any objective within research area 6.	AHRQ	1	625,000
		Education	2	729,398
		HRSA	1	100,000
		NIH	2	878,187
		NSF	2	393,237
Research area 7: Infrastructure and surveillance				
7.A	Conduct a needs assessment to determine how to merge or link administrative and/or surveillance databases that allow for tracking the involvement of people living with autism in health care, education, and social services by 2009.		No federal projects funded	
7.B	Conduct an annual "State of the States" assessment of existing state programs and supports for people and families living with autism by 2011.	CMS	2	540,491
7.C	Develop and have available to the research community a means by which to merge or link databases that allow for tracking the involvement of people in autism research by 2010.	NIH	1	2,040,353
7.D	Establish and maintain an international network of biobanks for the collection of brain tissue, fibroblasts for pluripotent stem cells, and other tissue or biological material, by acquisition sites that use standardized protocols for phenotyping, collection,	NIH	1	2,303,588

Table 1. (Continued)

Strategic Plan Research Area and Objectives[a]	Description of Objective	Agency	Number of Research Projects	Funds Awarded
	and regulated distribution of limited samples by 2011. This includes support for post-processing of tissue, such as genotyping, RNA expression profiling, and MRI. Protocols should be put into place to expand the capacities of ongoing large-scale children's studies to collect and store additional biomaterials, including newborn bloodspots, promoting detection of biological signatures. Support should also be provided to develop an international web-based digital brain atlas that would provide high-resolution 3-D images and quantitative anatomical data from tissue of patients with autism and disease controls across the lifespan, which could serve as an online resource for quantitative morphological studies, by 2014.			
7.E	Begin development of a web-based toolbox to assist researchers in effectively and responsibly disseminating their findings to the community, including people with autism, their families, and health practitioners, by 2011.	NIH	1	25,000
7.F	Create funding mechanisms that encourage rapid replication studies of novel or critical findings by 2011.		No federal projects funded	
7.G	Develop a web-based tool that provides population estimates of autism prevalence for States based on the most recent prevalence range and average identified by the Autism and Developmental Disabilities Monitoring Network by 2012.		No federal projects funded	

Strategic Plan Research Area and Objectives[a]	Description of Objective	Agency	Number of Research Projects	Funds Awarded
7.H	Create mechanisms to specifically support the contribution of data from 90 percent of newly initiated projects to the National Database for Autism Research, and link with other existing data resources by 2012.	NIH	6	9,583,653
7.I	Supplement existing Autism and Developmental Disabilities Monitoring Network sites to use population-based surveillance data to conduct at least five hypothesis-driven analyses evaluating factors that may contribute to changes in autism prevalence by 2012.	CDC	14	28,544,177
7.J	Develop the personnel and technical infrastructure to assist states, territories, and other countries that request assistance describing and investigating potential changes in the prevalence of autism and other developmental disabilities by 2013.	CDC	1	324,072
		NIH	1	150,000
7.K	Encourage programs and funding mechanisms that expand the research workforce, enhance interdisciplinary research training, and recruit early-career scientists into the autism field by 2013.	Education	3	1,457,164
		HRSA	1	2,868,488
		NIH	22	7,479,509
7.L	Expand the number of Autism and Developmental Disabilities Monitoring sites in order to conduct autism surveillance in children and adults; conduct complementary direct screening to inform completeness of ongoing surveillance; and expand efforts to include autism subtypes by 2015.	CDC	8	4,381,177

Table 1. (Continued)

Strategic Plan Research Area and Objectives[a]	Description of Objective	Agency	Number of Research Projects	Funds Awarded
7.M	Support 10 "Promising Practices" papers that describe innovative and successful services and supports being implemented in communities that benefit the full spectrum of people with autism, which can be replicated in other communities, by 2015.		No federal projects funded	
7.N	Enhance networks of clinical research sites offering clinical care in real-world settings that can collect and coordinate standardized and comprehensive diagnostic, biological (e.g., DNA, plasma, fibroblasts, urine), medical, and treatment history data that would provide a platform for conducting comparative effectiveness research and clinical trials of novel autism treatments by 2012.	HRSA	1	670,000
7.O	Create an information resource for autism researchers (e.g., PhenX Project) to share information to facilitate data sharing and standardization of methods across projects by 2013. This includes common protocols, instruments, designs, and other procedural documents, and should include updates on new technology and links to information on how to acquire and utilize technology in development. This can serve as a bidirectional information reference, with autism research driving the development of new resources and technologies, including new model systems, screening tools, and analytic techniques.	HRSA	1	2,142,000
		NIH	1	997,747

Strategic Plan Research Area and Objectives[a]	Description of Objective	Agency	Number of Research Projects	Funds Awarded
7.P	Provide resources to centers or facilities that develop promising vertebrate and invertebrate model systems, and make these models more easily available or expand the utility of current model systems, and support new approaches to develop high-throughput screening technologies to evaluate the validity of model systems by 2013.	NIH	1	1,588,780
7.Other	Not specific to any objective within research area 7.	NIH	34	52,663,973

Source: GAO analysis of data from the Interagency Autism Coordinating Committee (IACC) and federal agencies that funded autism research.

Notes: The number of autism research projects in the table reflects a project that HRSA broke-up into 7 sub-projects and categorized into different objectives for fiscal years 2010, 2011, and 2012. This project was not broken out in previous years; therefore, all funding for the project is attributed to objective 4.S.A for fiscal years 2008 and 2009. NIH jointly funded 1 autism research project with CDC and 1 project with EPA. These joint projects are counted separately in the total number of autism research projects for each of these agencies because the projects were awarded funding from different agencies. Additionally, from fiscal years 2008 through 2012, 6 autism projects were included in IACC data, but were categorized as "not specific to any research area," and 16 projects were not included in IACC data and, therefore, not categorized to the research areas. Furthermore, from fiscal years 2008 through 2011, CDC awarded funds for 9 research projects on autism and other developmental disabilities as part of its non-research autism-related activity, *Learn the Signs. Act Early.* CDC categorized the entire activity to the services research area; however, these 9 research projects are not included in the table because it was unclear if the individual research projects under *Learn the Signs. Act Early.* would also be categorized to the services research area. DOD's research projects include projects funded from DOD's fiscal years 2008 through 2011 appropriations. DOD's fiscal year 2012 appropriation for its medical research programs, including autism, was available for obligation through the end of fiscal year 2013—September 30, 2013. At the time of our review, DOD had not submitted data on its fiscal year 2012 research projects in response to OARC's request. As a result, the number of autism research projects for DOD does not include DOD's projects for fiscal year 2012.

When collecting and analyzing data, we included a project in the fiscal year in which it was awarded funds, even if funds remained available for obligation in future fiscal years—or, as is the case with DOD, the fiscal year of the appropriation from which the project or activity was awarded funds. For example, if a project was ongoing in another fiscal year, but did not receive an award in that year, we included the project in the fiscal year in which it received an award only. AHRQ and CMS each awarded one contract under which multiple autism-related projects were carried out. Education and SAMHSA also awarded contracts, of which an autism project was one component. Funding is not broken out in these contracts by project; therefore, the award amounts that we report for the AHRQ, CMS, Education, and SAMHSA autism projects under each contract are the agencies' estimates of the overall contract awards that were intended to support these projects.

[a]The strategic plan objective numbers are composed of the following components: the number indicates the strategic plan question, or research area, that the objective relates to; for strategic plan questions 1 through 6, the "S" and "L" indicate whether the objectives are short-term or long-term; and the final letter refers to the specific objective. Each of the 7 research areas includes an "Other" category. Although this category is not included in the strategic plan as an objective, it is used to categorize autism research that relates to a specific research area, but not a specific objective.

APPENDIX IV: AGENCIES' NON-RESEARCH AUTISM-RELATED ACTIVITIES, FISCAL YEARS 2008 THROUGH 2011

Five agencies funded non-research autism-related activities from fiscal year 2008 through 2011—Administration for Community Living (ACL), Centers for Disease Control and Prevention (CDC), Department of Defense (DOD), Department of Education (Education), and Health Resources and Services Administration (HRSA). The agencies funded activities that we categorized by the following activity type: awareness campaign, information dissemination, training, and other types of activities. This appendix includes a list of each activity, by agency and by activity type. Also included is the amount of funding awarded by the agency—that was related to autism—under each activity between fiscal years 2008 and 2011; as well as a brief description of the primary purpose, strategy for achieving that purpose, and target population of each activity.[1]

ACL: Information Dissemination Activity

Autism NOW: National Autism Resource and Information Center

- Funding: $2.6 million
- Purpose: Gather, organize, and provide diverse stakeholders with readily accessible, high-quality resources and information related to community-based services that support independent living and self-determination, treatment protocols that promote community-based experiences (e.g., education, employment, recreation, transportation, early intervention, and child care), and evidence-based interventions.
- Strategy: Website provides information and links to resources related to four main components: (1) at home, (2) on the job, (3) in the classroom, and (4) in the community. The website also offers webinars and blogs on various topics related to autism and other developmental disabilities.
- Target Population: Individuals with autism and other developmental disabilities, their families, and other targeted stakeholders concerned with autism.

CDC: Awareness Campaign/Information Dissemination Activity

Learn the Signs. Act Early

- Funding: $9.8 million[2]
- Purpose: Improve early identification of children with autism and other developmental disabilities so children and families can get the services and support they need as early as possible.
- Strategy: The program is made up of three components: (1) the health education campaign promotes awareness of healthy developmental milestones in early childhood, the importance of tracking each child's development, and the importance of acting early if there are concerns; (2) the Act Early Initiative works with state, territorial, and national partners to improve early childhood systems by enhancing collaborative efforts to improve screening and referral to early intervention services, and to promote *Learn the Signs. Act Early.* messages and tools, and improve early identification efforts in their states and territories; and (3) the research and evaluation component improves campaign materials and implementation activities, and increases the understanding of the factors that influence early identification and referral.
- Target Population: Parents, early educators, and health care providers.

DOD: Information Dissemination Activity

Extension & Military Partnership Autism Project

- Funding: $1.3 million
- Purpose: Assessment of educational services for children with autism, emotional/behavioral disorders, and intellectual disabilities near military installations; and national review of best practices around educational support for children with the identified disabilities. Data is used to update the current online Education Directory for Children with Special Needs, which provides assignment personnel and families of military dependents with information they need to make informed assignment decisions.
- Strategy: Website consists of two main components that provide tools and resources to help with the transition to a new military installation: (1) the Early Intervention Directory focuses on early intervention services for children from birth to 3 years old; and (2) the School-Age

Directory focuses on education services for children with special needs, 3 to 21 years of age.

- Target Population: Military families, who have children with autism or other developmental disabilities, using educational services in selected states.

Education: Training Activities

Personnel Development to Improve Services and Results for Children with Disabilities

- Funding: $42.4 million
- Purpose: To help address state-identified needs for highly qualified personnel by preparing personnel in special education, related services, early intervention, and regular education to work with children with disabilities; and to ensure that those personnel have the skills and knowledge—derived from practices that have been determined through research and experience to be successful—needed to serve these children. This could include preparing personnel to work with children with autism and their families.
- Strategy: This activity supports two types of personnel preparation projects. (1) Projects designed to prepare special education early intervention, or related services personnel to serve as higher education faculty and researchers. These projects culminate in a doctoral degree or provide postdoctoral learning opportunities. (2) Projects designed to prepare special education, early intervention, or related services, direct service providers or administrators to work in state educational agencies, lead agencies, local educational agencies, early intervention services programs, or schools. They culminate in a baccalaureate, master's, education specialist, or doctoral degree; or state certification, endorsement, or licensure. The projects may provide specialization in conducting autism research or providing services for children with autism and their families.
- Target Population: Scholars in special education, early intervention, and related services programs.

Personnel Development to Improve Services and Results for Children with Disabilities; National Professional Development Center on Autism Spectrum Disorders

- Funding: $4 million
- Purpose: Provides resources, professional development, and technical assistance to help address state-identified needs for highly qualified personnel in special education, related services, early intervention, and regular education to work with infants, toddlers, and children with disabilities; and ensure that those personnel have the necessary skills and knowledge, derived from practices that have been determined through scientifically based research and experience, to be successful in serving those children.
- Strategy: The project goals are organized around four content areas: (1) content development, (2) professional development, (3) technical assistance, and (4) evaluation. Content development involves translating information about evidence-based practices— or educational interventions—for children with autism into resources for service providers. Professional development entails providing training to state professional development providers and practitioners, as well as establishing training sites that model evidence-based practices in participating states. Technical assistance includes providing ongoing site-based training and establishing a network of professional development sites, trainees, and professional consultants. Evaluation involves collecting follow-up data on the use of evidence-based practices, practitioner skills, and child and family outcomes.
- Target Population: States' departments of education receiving funds under Part B and state lead agencies under Part C of the Individuals with Disabilities Education Act, and those that they provide professional development to, such as teachers and practitioners who serve individuals from birth through 21 years of age with autism.[3]

State Personnel Development Grants Program

- Funding: $6.5 million
- Purpose: Assist state educational agencies in reforming and improving their systems for personnel preparation and professional development in early intervention, education, and transition services in order to improve results for children with disabilities.
- Strategy: Supports implementation of a State Personnel Development Plan. This plan must identify and address the state and local needs for

the personnel preparation and professional development of personnel, as well as individuals who provide direct supplementary aids and services to children with disabilities. The projects must use evidence-based professional development practices that will increase implementation of evidence-based practices and result in improved outcomes for children with disabilities; provide ongoing assistance to personnel receiving professional development that supports the implementation of evidence-based practices; and use technology to more efficiently and effectively provide ongoing professional development to personnel, including to personnel in rural areas and to other populations, such as personnel in urban or high-need local educational agencies.

- Target Population: State educational agencies in the 50 states, the District of Columbia, the Commonwealth of Puerto Rico, Guam, Virgin Islands, American Samoa, and the Commonwealth of the Northern Mariana Islands that have a State Personnel Development Plan and those personnel they train, such as teachers, administrators, and early intervention providers.

Rehabilitation Continuing Education Program

- Funding: $2.8 million
- Purpose: This program is designed to ensure that skilled personnel are available to serve the rehabilitation needs of individuals with disabilities. It is also designed to provide support to the public vocational rehabilitation system; provide advice, technical support, and training to the state vocational rehabilitation agencies and their community partners.
- Strategy: There are 10 regional Technical Assistance and Continuing Education centers that serve either a federal region or another geographical area and provide for a broad integrated sequence of training activities that focus on meeting recurrent and common training needs of employed rehabilitation personnel throughout a multi-state geographical area. One center has developed materials to train vocational rehabilitation staff on autism. These materials are made available to other Technical Assistance and Continuing Education centers and to state vocational rehabilitation agencies for staff training purposes.
- Target Population: State vocational rehabilitation agencies and the professionals they train.

Education: Other Activity Types

Developing Hispanic-Serving Institutions Program-Title V

- Funding: $0.3 million
- Purpose: To assist Hispanic-serving institutions to expand educational opportunities for, and improve the attainment of, Hispanic students. It also enables these institutions to expand and enhance their academic offerings, program quality, and institutional stability.
- Strategy: Activities supported include: scientific or laboratory equipment for teaching; construction or renovation of instructional facilities; faculty development; purchase of educational materials; academic tutoring or counseling programs; funds and administrative management; joint use of facilities; endowment funds; distance learning academic instruction; teacher education; and student support services.
- Target Population: Hispanic students and the postsecondary institutions that serve them.

Fund for the Improvement of Education

- Funding: $1.6 million
- Purpose: To support nationally significant programs to improve the quality of elementary and secondary education at the state and local levels, and help all students meet challenging state academic content standards and student achievement standards.
- Strategy: Types of projects funded include activities to promote systemic education reform at the state and local levels, including scientifically based research, development, and evaluation designed to improve student academic achievement at the state and local levels; and strategies for effective parent and community involvement.
- Target Population: Students

Fund for the Improvement of Postsecondary Education Congressionally Directed Projects

- Funding: $1.4 million
- Purpose: Address critical national needs and support Education's mission of increasing access to quality postsecondary education.
- Strategy: These are noncompetitive grants that Education manages pursuant to Congress' direction to provide such grants to certain recipients for specified purposes and in specified amounts.

- Target Population: Individuals or institutions involved in or impacted by postsecondary education.

Technology and Media Services for Individuals with Disabilities program: Steppingstones of Technology Innovation for Children with Disabilities

- Funding: $1.0 million
- Purpose: (1) Improve results for children with disabilities by promoting the development, demonstration, and use of technology; (2) support educational media service activities designed to be of educational value in the classroom setting to children with disabilities; and (3) provide support for captioning and video description that are appropriate for use in the classroom setting.
- Strategy: Develop, implement, and evaluate innovative technology approaches designed to improve results for children with disabilities. Phase 1 projects must develop, refine, and test the feasibility of specific technology-based approaches. Phase 2 projects must subject technology-based approaches to rigorous field-based research to determine their effectiveness.
- Target Population: Children served under the Individuals with Disabilities Education Act, including children with autism.

HRSA: Training Activities

Developmental-Behavioral Pediatrics Training Program

- Funding: $7.3 million
- Purpose: The primary goal is to train the next generation of leaders in developmental-behavioral pediatrics; and provide pediatric practitioners, residents, and medical students with essential biopsychosocial knowledge and clinical expertise. The program also supports continuing education for pediatricians and other providers to implement evidence-based interventions for autism and other developmental disabilities.
- Strategy: The 3-year program curriculum includes course work and clinical exposure to psychosocial and biological sciences, growth and development, adaptation, injury prevention, disease prevention, and health promotion. Projects are also encouraged to cosponsor, with child psychiatry, an ongoing Collaborative Office Rounds group as a

training experience for fellows and a continuing education experience for community providers. Grantees also provide continuing education activities for practicing physicians and are encouraged to offer technical assistance and consultation to pediatric residency training programs so that they can improve their own developmental-behavioral program components.

- Target Population: Fellows in developmental-behavioral pediatrics preparing for leadership roles as teachers, investigators, and clinicians advancing the field of developmental-behavioral pediatrics; pediatric practitioners, residents, and medical students.

Leadership Education in Neurodevelopmental and Other Related Disabilities (LEND) Training Program

- Funding: $107.2 million
- Purpose: Improve the health of children who have, or are at risk for developing, neurodevelopmental and other related disabilities by providing high quality interdisciplinary graduate leadership training to child health professionals from diverse backgrounds and preparing those professionals to assume leadership roles. This includes supporting the training of individuals who can provide screening, diagnostic evaluation, and evidence-based interventions for autism and other developmental disabilities.
- Strategy: Provides interdisciplinary leadership training and encourages providers to think holistically about the needs of children with autism and other developmental disabilities, as well as their families. The training curriculum includes graduate education at the master's, doctoral, and postdoctoral training levels, with an emphasis on developing a knowledge and experience base that includes: (1) knowledge of all aspects of neurodevelopmental and related disabilities, including autism; (2) acquisition of interdisciplinary team skills; and (3) knowledge of the family environment and cultural competency.
- Target Population: Trainees are individuals working toward a graduate degree across 14 disciplines—including medicine, dentistry, psychology, social work, nutrition, language and motor therapies, audiology, genetics, health administration, special education, and nursing—or are enrolled in a postgraduate program with an emphasis on infants, children, and adolescents with special health care needs. Trainees show promise to become leaders in the material and child

health field in the areas of teaching, research, clinical practice, and/or administration and policymaking.

National Combating Autism Interdisciplinary Training Resource Center

- Funding: $2.5 million
- Purpose: Improve the health of children who have, or are at risk for developing, autism and other developmental disabilities by providing technical assistance to LEND and Developmental-Behavioral Pediatrics grantees to better train professionals to utilize valid and reliable screening tools for diagnosing or ruling out autism and provide evidence-based interventions for children.
- Strategy: The center supports LEND and Developmental-Behavioral Pediatrics grantees by providing technical assistance, disseminating information and resources, and providing program coordination to promote collaboration across the grantees.
- Target Population: LEND and Developmental-Behavioral Pediatrics grantees.

HRSA: Other Activity Types

State Implementation and Planning Grants

- Funding: $11.8 million
- Purpose: Improve access to comprehensive, coordinated health care and related services by implementing state plans to improve the system of services.
- Strategy: Although the plans vary widely by state, common elements include a focus on partnerships between professionals and families of children and youth with autism; access to a culturally competent family-centered medical home; access to adequate health insurance and financing of services; early and continuous screening for autism and other developmental disabilities; community services organized for easy use by families; and transition services for youth entering adult health care.
- Target Population: States with an existing plan for improving the system of services for children with autism and developmental disabilities.

State Public Health Coordinating Center

- Funding: $1.1 million
- Purpose: Improve the health of children who have, or are at risk for developing, autism and other developmental disabilities.
- Strategy: Coordinating with the state implementation and planning grantees and developing a strategy for defining, supporting, and monitoring the role of state public health agencies in assuring early and timely identification, diagnosis, and intervention.
- Target Population: State implementation and planning grantees, and broader state public health programs.

End Notes

[1] CDC has recently reported 2 estimates of autism prevalence: 1 in 88 and 1 in 50 children in the United States have been identified as having autism. According to CDC, there are several differences between the 2 studies used to determine the estimates that can contribute to the differing results, such as the population covered, method of data collection, and time periods covered. CDC reported its estimate of 1 in 88 in March 2012, which was based on reviews of health and education records of children 8 years of age residing in 14 select population-based sites in the United States during calendar year 2008. The estimate of 1 in 50 was reported in March 2013 and was based on parent reports of a past diagnosis in a representative national sample of children 6 to 17 years of age in calendar years 2011 and 2012. CDC views the 2 data collection methods and estimates to be complementary. According to CDC, each provides unique supplemental information on the population of children with autism. Prior to these recent estimates, in 2009, CDC reported an estimated prevalence of 1 in 110 children in the United States, which was based on data from calendar year 2006.

[2] In this report, we use the term "autism" to refer to autism spectrum disorder as defined in the fourth edition of the *Diagnostic and Statistical Manual of Mental Disorders*, which was effective during the time period covered by our review. American Psychiatric Association, *Diagnostic and Statistical Manual of Mental Disorders*, 4th Edition, Text Revision (DSM-IV-TR) (Arlington, VA: American Psychiatric Association, 2000).

[3] These agencies are the Department of Defense; Department of Education; Environmental Protection Agency; National Science Foundation; and eight agencies within HHS—Administration for Children and Families, Administration for Community Living, Agency for Healthcare Research and Quality, CDC, Centers for Medicare & Medicaid Services, Health Resources and Services Administration, National Institutes of Health, and Substance Abuse and Mental Health Services Administration.

[4] "Autism-related activities" include agency activities that are specific to autism as well as agency activities that are not autism-specific, but through which a project that was autism-specific or had an autism-specific component was funded.

[5] Pub. L. No. 109-416, 120 Stat. 2821 (Dec. 19, 2006). These activities were reauthorized and funding was authorized to be appropriated through fiscal year 2014 under the Combating Autism Reauthorization Act of 2011. Pub. L. No. 112-32, 125 Stat. 361 (Sept. 30, 2011).

We previously reported on HHS agencies' response to the CAA. See GAO, *Combating Autism Act: HHS Agencies Responded with New and Continuing Activities, Including Oversight,* GAO-13-232 (Washington, D.C. Feb. 27, 2013).

[6] Pub. L. No. 106-310, § 104, 114 Stat. 1101, 1109 (Oct. 17, 2000).

[7] IACC membership as of November 2013.

[8] The CAA also requires the IACC to develop and annually update a summary of advances in autism research; and to make recommendations to the Secretary of Health and Human Services regarding any appropriate changes to federal autism activities, including recommendations with respect to the strategic plan on autism research and recommendations regarding public participation in decisions relating to autism.

[9] A cooperative agreement is an alternative assistance instrument used instead of a grant whenever substantial federal involvement with the recipient during performance is anticipated.

[10] We initially collected data directly from the individual federal agencies regarding the autism research and autism-related activities that were awarded funds from fiscal years 2008 to 2011. While our work was in progress, in January 2013, we learned that OARC, on behalf of the IACC, had started collecting data on research projects funded by federal agencies in fiscal years 2011 and 2012. We opted to include the fiscal year 2012 research projects that agencies reported to OARC. We relied on the agency data we collected on the non-research activities awarded between fiscal years 2008 and 2011. Also, DOD's fiscal year 2012 appropriation for its medical research programs, including autism, was available for obligation through the end of fiscal year 2013—September 30, 2013. At the time of our review, DOD had not submitted data on its fiscal year 2012 research projects in response to OARC's request. As a result, our report does not include data on DOD's fiscal year 2012 autism research.

[11] See for example, GAO, *2013 Annual Report: Actions Needed to Reduce Fragmentation, Overlap, and Duplication and Achieve Other Financial Benefits*, GAO-13-279SP (Washington, D.C.: Apr. 9, 2013) and GAO, *2012 Annual Report: Opportunities to Reduce Duplication, Overlap, and Fragmentation, Achieve Savings, and Enhance Revenue,* GAO-12-342SP (Washington, D.C.: Feb. 28, 2012).

[12] We interviewed eight federal members of the IACC. We did not interview officials from two agencies that are members of the IACC—the Administration for Children and Families (ACF) and the Food and Drug Administration. ACF awarded funds for one autism-related research project in fiscal year 2012. The Food and Drug Administration did not fund any autism research or autism-related activities during the time frame of our review. We also did not interview Substance Abuse and Mental Health Services Administration (SAMHSA) officials. SAMHSA is not a member of the IACC, but awarded funds for one autism-related research project in fiscal year 2011. We selected six nonfederal members to interview; however, in July 2013, one of the nonfederal members we interviewed stepped down from the IACC.

[13] See, for example, GAO, *Managing for Results: Key Considerations for Implementing Interagency Collaborative Mechanisms*, GAO-12-1022 (Washington, D.C.: Sept. 27, 2012); GAO, *Results-Oriented Government: Practices That Can Help Enhance and Sustain Collaboration among Federal Agencies,* GAO-06-15 (Washington, D.C.: Oct. 21, 2005); and GAO, *Standards for Internal Control in the Federal Government*, GAO/AIMD-00-21.3.1 (Washington, D.C.: November 1999).

[14] A developmental disability is a chronic condition caused by mental impairment, physical impairment, or both that begins any time during prenatal development up to age 22 and

usually persists throughout a person's life. Individuals with developmental disabilities have substantial functional limitations in at least 3 major life activities such as language, mobility, learning, self-help, and independent living. Developmental disabilities may include cerebral palsy, hearing loss, intellectual disability, and impaired vision.

[15] See HHS, OARC, NIH, *Report to Congress on Activities Related to Autism Spectrum Disorder and Other Developmental Disabilities Under the Combating Autism Act of 2006 (FY 2006 – FY 2009)* (Rockville, Md.: December 2010, revised April 2011). According to OARC officials, OARC will be preparing another report to Congress on autism activities as required by the reauthorization of the CAA. This report is expected to be submitted to Congress by the Secretary of Health and Human Services and then released to the public in the fall of 2013.

[16] AHRQ and DOD were not members of the IACC when the CAA was enacted in 2006, but have joined since the act's reauthorization in 2011. ACL was created in 2012. Prior to this, the component of ACL that funded an autism activity was part of ACF and a previous IACC member. SAMHSA was also a previous IACC member.

[17] ACL did not fund autism research from fiscal year 2008 through fiscal year 2012; ACL funded one non-research autism-related activity during this time period.

[18] Principal investigators are typically individuals designated by the applicant organization, such as a university, to have the appropriate level of authority and responsibility to direct the project or program to be supported by the award. A funding opportunity announcement is a publicly available document in which a federal agency makes known its intentions to award discretionary grants or cooperative agreements, usually as a result of competition for funds. Funding opportunity announcements may be known as program announcements, requests for applications, notices of funding availability, solicitations, or other names depending on the agency and type of program. A request for proposal is a type of mechanism used to solicit proposals for a contract.

[19] NIH and other HHS agencies have developed omnibus parent announcements for use by investigators who wish to submit investigator-initiated research.

[20] Another such required report is a summary of advances in autism research, which annually lists and summarizes the findings of autism research publications that the IACC deems to have significantly advanced the field.

[21] Six research areas have separate short- and long-term objectives. For one research area—infrastructure and surveillance—the IACC considers all objectives within that area to be both short- and long-term objectives.

[22] The 2009 strategic plan contained 6 questions and 40 objectives. The question—"What other infrastructure and surveillance needs must be met?"—as well as additional objectives were added to the 2010 strategic plan. During the IACC's most recent update of the strategic plan—the 2012 update—the IACC did not review or change the number of objectives, but instead summarized the new advances and opportunities in the field under each of the 7 research areas. Therefore, the most recent plan that contains the research areas and objectives is the 2011 strategic plan.

[23] The first portfolio analysis—the 2008 portfolio analysis—which contains information on research funded in 2008, was published in April 2010. The 2009 portfolio analysis was published in June 2011. The most recent portfolio analysis—the 2010 portfolio analysis—was published in July 2012.

[24] We consider reports and other information that are prepared by OARC, on behalf of the IACC, to be IACC information.

[25] The web tool, accessed August 27, 2013, is available at https://iacc.hhs.gov/apps/ portfolio-analysis-web-tool/projects.

[26] For our analysis, we determined the average number of IACC full committee meetings from calendar years 2008 through 2012. In addition to these meetings, the IACC subcommittees have met, and the IACC has held town hall gatherings, scientific workshops, and planning workgroup meetings. There are two IACC subcommittees. The subcommittee for basic and translational research supports IACC activities related to biomedical and behavioral research, research collaborations and resources, and other related issues. The subcommittee for services research and policy supports IACC activities related to service research and service policy, including service provision, service research, access, housing, transition, social inclusion, health disparities, healthcare costs, the Patient Protection and Affordable Care Act, and safety issues.

[27] See, for example, GAO-13-279SP and GAO-12-342SP.

[28] Grants.gov serves as the central grant identification and application portal for more than 1,000 federal grant programs that fund approximately $500 billion in grants from 26 grant-making agencies for activities such as training, research, planning, construction; and the provision of services in areas such as health care, education, transportation, and homeland security. See http://www.grants.gov, accessed August 26, 2013. ClinicalTrials.gov is a resource for information about clinical research studies, also referred to as clinical trials. It includes information on federally funded and non-federally funded studies. See http://www.clinicaltrials.gov, accessed August 26, 2013.

[29] See, for example, GAO-12-1022 and GAO, *Managing for Results: Critical Issues for Improving Federal Agencies' Strategic Plans*, GAO/GGD-97-180 (Washington, D.C.: Sept. 16, 1997).

[30] GAO-06-15 and GAO/AIMD-00-21.3.1.

[31] We found that 84 percent of projects were potentially duplicative by identifying the number of projects that were categorized to the same strategic plan objective and funded by different agencies. For those projects that were not categorized to a specific objective, but were categorized to one of the 7 research areas, we identified the number of projects that were categorized to the same research area and funded by different agencies. We summed the projects identified and compared the results to the total number of research projects funded during the time period of our review. Our findings suggest the potential for, but not actual, duplication. We could not assess 31 projects for duplication. NIH categorized 6 of its research projects as not relating to any of the research areas. Additionally, 16 research projects were not included in IACC data. Furthermore, from fiscal years 2008 through 2011, CDC awarded funds for 9 research projects on autism and other developmental disabilities as part of its non-research autism-related activity, *Learn the Signs. Act Early.* CDC categorized the entire activity to the services research area; however, we did not categorize these 9 research projects to the same objective because it was unclear if the individual research projects under *Learn the Signs. Act Early.* would also be categorized to the services research area.

[32] According to OARC officials, the strategic plan objectives represent gap areas that need additional attention or emphasis, and are not meant to cover all areas of autism research; therefore, research projects that are categorized to a research area, but not a specific objective, focus on research outside of the specific gap areas represented in the strategic plan.

[33] During the course of our review, we learned that HRSA, AHRQ, and Education funded reviews of evidence regarding the effectiveness of autism interventions for children and adolescents.

Using the framework established in our previous work on duplication, we obtained additional data from these agencies that allowed us to determine if there was duplication by comparing the projects' purposes, strategies, and target populations.

[34] A systematic review is a critical assessment and evaluation of all research studies that address a particular clinical issue.

[35] Education's project published a report of its findings in 2010, and the AHRQ project published its report in 2011.

[36] Although CDC's *Learn the Signs. Act Early.* campaign is generally a non-research autism-related activity, one institution received funding from CDC through this campaign to conduct research on autism and other developmental disabilities. We included the funds awarded to this institution for research as research in our analysis.

[37] The Autism Research Program Integration Panel is comprised of experts and leaders in the field, including doctors, scientists, and consumers. It recommends the office's autism research priorities and recommends projects to be funded annually.

[38] We asked agency officials about the extent to which they used the strategic plan and portfolio analysis. The agencies that do not regularly use these documents are ACL, AHRQ, Education, EPA, and NSF. While AHRQ does not regularly use these documents, AHRQ officials stated that they consulted the IACC when developing their systematic reviews related to autism. Additionally, CMS officials stated that while they do not use the portfolio analysis, the autism research projects they funded resulted from strategic plan objectives, among other things, such as the general rise of autism and CMS's own initiative and interest in providing information to the professionals who work with CMS. In addition, HRSA officials stated they used the strategic plan when first creating their autism activities and on an ongoing basis. Officials stated that they included language in their autism funding opportunity announcements about their interest in intervention research, underserved populations, and other broad areas noted as gaps in the strategic plan; however, HRSA officials made no mention of using the portfolio analysis.

[39] In its comments on a draft of this report, Education stated that after holding a meeting with OARC officials in August 2013, it determined that its research related to interventions could be categorized to the strategic plan; subsequently, it has categorized those projects accordingly.

[40] The portfolio analysis and web tool indicate whether an objective has been fulfilled based on the funding of projects related to that objective in a given year and annualized funding goals for each objective set by the IACC.

[41] The guidance states that project information should only be provided if a project relates to evaluating training for service providers. Projects that solely involved the administration of services were not to be provided.

[42] The DOD Air Force study, *Comprehensive Clinical Phenotyping and Genetic Mapping for the Discovery of Autism Susceptibility Genes,* was conducted with the Research Institute at Nationwide Children's Hospital in Ohio and awarded funds in 2008 and 2009.

[43] The Education study, *Combining Technologies to Maximize Outcomes: Telemedicine and Online Training Program for Parents of Children with Autism*, was awarded funds in 2008.

[44] The most recent portfolio analysis is described as including information on autism research funded by major federal agencies. The portfolio analysis also includes information on autism research funded by certain nonfederal organizations.

[45] In prior work, we established certain key features that benefit collaborative mechanisms (see GAO-12-1022).

[46] GAO/AIMD-00-21.3.1.

[47] For example, while 1 objective recommended launching 3 projects related to underlying biological pathways of genetic conditions related to autism, 72 projects were funded from fiscal year 2008 through 2012.

[48] According to OARC officials, the web tool will also be released in the first quarter of calendar year 2014. At the time of our review, OARC officials were not certain whether the portfolio analysis would include 2011 and 2012 data combined or separated; however, they stated that the web tool would report the data separately, similar to the presentation of prior years' data.

[49] GAO-06-15.

[50] We found some other instances where an agency funded another agency to conduct research or other activities through an interagency agreement or memorandum of understanding; however, the projects were not co-managed.

[51] See for example, GAO-13-279SP and GAO-12-342SP.

[52] See federal internal control standard for information and communications. GAO/AIMD-00-21.3.1.

[53] In addition, NIH officials stated that, before awarding funding, NIH program and grants management staff are to ensure that there is no budgetary, scientific, or commitment overlap by reviewing documentation of "other support" identified by the applicant (which includes all financial resources, whether federal, nonfederal, commercial or organizational, available in direct support of an individual's research endeavors, including, but not limited to, research grants, cooperative agreements, contracts, or organizational awards, but not training awards, prizes, or gifts). Officials from AHRQ, DOD, Education, and NSF also told us they rely on similar disclosure from applicants.

[54] Project officers are agency officials that are responsible for managing and overseeing grants.

[55] Our prior work identified limitations in the ability of DOD and NIH to readily access comprehensive medical research information funded by other agencies. See GAO-12-342SP. DOD officials stated that DOD and NIH are working together to address these concerns. Specifically, NIH has provided a DOD official with access to an NIH database that contains information about certain funded health research projects. According to DOD officials, they intend to begin expanding this effort to all programs funded by DOD's Office of Congressionally Directed Medical Research Programs in the beginning of calendar year 2014, but could not provide specifics on when it would be expanded to autism research.

[56] See HHS, OARC, NIH, *Report to Congress on Activities Related to Autism Spectrum Disorder and Other Developmental Disabilities Under the Combating Autism Act of 2006 (FY 2006 – FY 2009)* (Rockville, Md.: December 2010, revised April 2011).

End Notes for Appendix I

[1] We interviewed federal members of the IACC, with the exception of Administration for Children and Families (ACF) and the Food and Drug Administration. ACF awarded funds for one autism-related project in fiscal year 2012. The Food and Drug Administration did not fund any autism-related projects during the time frame of our review. We selected six nonfederal members to interview; however, in July 2013, one of the nonfederal members we interviewed stepped down from the IACC.

[2] A cooperative agreement is an alternative assistance instrument used instead of a grant whenever substantial federal involvement with the recipient during performance is anticipated.

[3] When collecting and analyzing data, we included a research project or a non-research autism-related activity in the fiscal year in which it was awarded funds—even if funds remained available for obligation in future fiscal years—or, as is the case with the Department of Defense, the fiscal year of the appropriation from which the project or activity was awarded funds. For example, if a research project was ongoing in another fiscal year, but did not receive an award in that year, we included the project in the fiscal year in which it received an award only. The Agency for Healthcare Research and Quality (AHRQ) and Centers for Medicare & Medicaid Services (CMS) each awarded one contract under which multiple autism-related projects were conducted. The Department of Education (Education) and Substance Abuse and Mental Health Services Administration (SAMHSA) also awarded contracts of which an autism project was one component. Funding is not broken out in these contracts by research project; therefore, the award amounts that we report for the AHRQ, CMS, Education, and SAMHSA autism projects under each contract are the agencies' estimates of the amount of the overall contract awards that was intended to support these projects or activities.

[4] We counted a project once if the project had the same project number unless the title changed. If the project title changed during the time of our review period, we confirmed that the project start dates were the same. If the start dates were the same, we considered the project to be the same and counted it once. If the project start dates were different, we counted the project as a separate project. If the project start date was not available, we looked to see if other distinguishing characteristics, such as project description, were similar. We did not count a project as a "new" or "separate" project if the project received a new award for another project period—the total period for which support of a project has been programmatically approved. For example, a principal investigator may submit a competing continuation application to continue the project after the initial project period. In addition, the National Institutes of Health (NIH) supports discrete projects performed by investigators in their specific area of interest. It also supports organized efforts of several principal investigators conducting related research projects. In this latter case, we counted each project run by a separate principal investigator as a separate project.

[5] For example, if the portfolio analysis included a project number not in the list provided by the agency, we inquired with the agency whether the project was autism-specific or had an autism-specific component and should therefore be included in our review. We obtained fiscal years 2009 and 2010 data online via the web tool. For fiscal year 2008, we obtained the portfolio analysis data from the Office of Autism Research Coordination.

[6] We initially collected data directly from the individual federal agencies on their autism research and autism-related activities for which funds were awarded from fiscal years 2008 to 2011. We opted to include the fiscal year 2012 research projects that agencies reported to OARC. We relied on the agency data we collected on the non-research activities awarded between fiscal years 2008 and 2011.

[7] Over the years, OARC has changed its guidance on the types of projects to include in the portfolio analysis. The most recent guidance has more narrow criteria than past years, but since we reviewed data from multiple years, overall, the criteria was different.

[8] If supplemental awards were categorized differently from the base project in the same year, we counted them as separate projects.

[9] As part of its analysis for the portfolio analysis and web tool, OARC reviews the agency submissions and can change the strategic plan question and objective categorization if it thinks that a project should be categorized differently for consistency and accuracy purposes. At the time of our review, OARC had not conducted its analysis of some of the agencies' fiscal year 2011 and 2012 data. Therefore, some of the projects in our review may be categorized to the strategic plan research areas and objectives differently than in the forthcoming fiscal year 2011 and 2012 portfolio analysis and web tool. This applies to approximately 34 projects. In addition, in its comments on a draft of this report, Education stated that, in August 2013, OARC and Education officials held a meeting to clarify the terms used to categorize projects. As a result, Education changed the categorization of select projects; however, Education officials stated that these changes would not have a material effect on this report.

[10] Projects may have been categorized to the strategic plan questions and objectives differently over time. According to OARC officials, this is mainly due to more objectives being added to the strategic plan as well as improved accuracy in the categorization by agencies. Because we are using the most recent fiscal year's strategic plan question and objective categories, all of the funding for a project will be attributed to that category, regardless of whether the project was categorized differently in previous years.

[11] See for example, GAO-13-279SP and GAO-12-342SP.

End Notes for Appendix III

[1] Twelve agencies were included in the scope of our review. However, the Administration for Community Living (ACL) did not fund autism research from fiscal year 2008 through fiscal year 2012. ACL funded one non-research autism-related activity during this time period and so it is not discussed in this appendix.

End Notes for Appendix IV

[1] Most of Education's activities included projects that were not related to autism. The funding presented for Education represents the funding amounts that supported projects, under each activity, that were autism-specific or had a component to them that was autism-specific. CDC funded one non-research activity—*Learn the Signs. Act Early.* between fiscal years 2008 and 2011. The funding amount for *Learn the Signs. Act Early.* reflects funding to support contracts and cooperative agreements, as well as activities conducted internally at the agency, such as funding for staffing and personnel costs.

[2] This funding amount reflects CDC's total funding for *Learn the Signs. Act Early.*, with the exception of research funded under this activity—totaling approximately $1.7 million.

[3] The Individuals with Disabilities Education Act is a federal law that provides federal funds on a formula grant basis to assist states in providing early intervention, special education, and related services to eligible children with disabilities. Part B of the act is a program administered by state educational agencies to make a free appropriate public education available to children with disabilities beginning at age 3, and potentially until age 22, depending on state law or practice.

Part C of the act is a program administered by a lead agency in a state to make available early intervention services to infants and toddlers with disabilities from birth until age 3, and their families.

INDEX

C

D

E

F

G

H

I

P

Q

R

U

V

W

Y